MY JOURNEY

Losing 40 Lbs. in 4 Months While over 40

TANAE WALKER

Publishing assistance provided by TJS Publishing House, www.tonyajoyner.com

Cover Art Photo: Todd Walker of TNT Productions
Cover Art Hair: LaTasha Newman at Salon K
Make-up: Tanae Walker

Published in the United States of America
ISBN-13: 978-0-578-51580-9
ISBN-10: 0-578-51580-6

DEDICATION

I would like to first dedicate this book to my father, Robert C Jones! He instilled in me the importance of healthy eating and working out. I thoroughly enjoyed us working out at the gym over my summers off from teaching. He was my first drill sergeant whipping me into shape! He also encouraged me to write this book on how I lost the weight in such a short amount of time. Love you, Daddy!

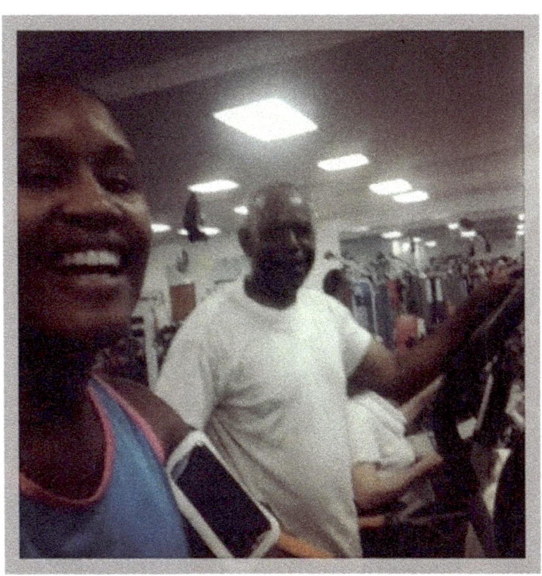

DEDICATION

I would be remiss if I didn't mention my dear, loving, caring and supportive husband, Todd Walker! He was there from the beginning of this journey when I was crying while I stared unbelievingly at the scale at the gym. We were each other's accountability partner. He would challenge me to run when I so dearly wanted to walk. I can still hear him yell the feet cadences in my mind. "Left, Left, Left-Right-Left" as we ran around our neighborhood. He always pushed me to reach new limits and goals in my weight loss journey. He has loved me unconditionally when I was obese and even now at my healthiest of weights. Love you, Baby!

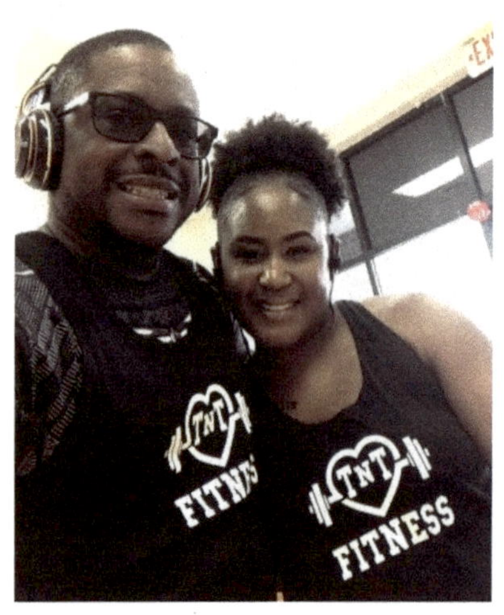

DEDICATION

I also would like to thank my Father-in-law, Earl! He always had suggestions for healthy foods I should try and foods that I should avoid. When it became obvious I had lost 30 pounds, he suggested that I write a book. He also mentioned that I should promote and create workout videos as well. It was like he was reading my mind! Thank you, Earl, for believing in me, and that I could and would write this book!

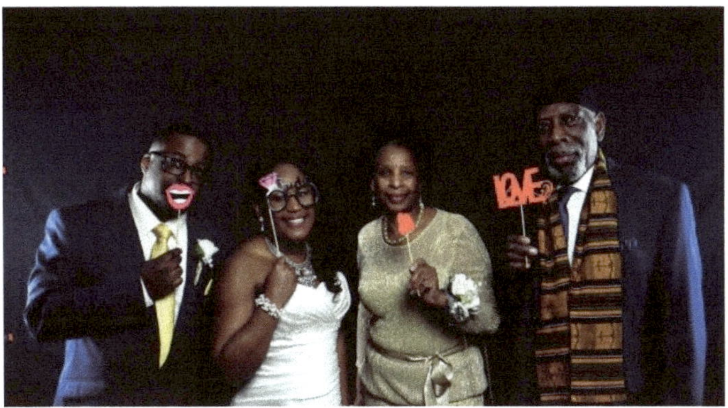

DEDICATION

I would not have this opportunity to become an author without the sacrifice of my ancestors before me. Even though at that time enslaved African- Americans were forbidden to read and write, Mrs. Wheatley persevered and had her first book published in England. Her later books were finally published in the United States. I dedicate this book also to Phyllis Wheatley who was the first African American published author.

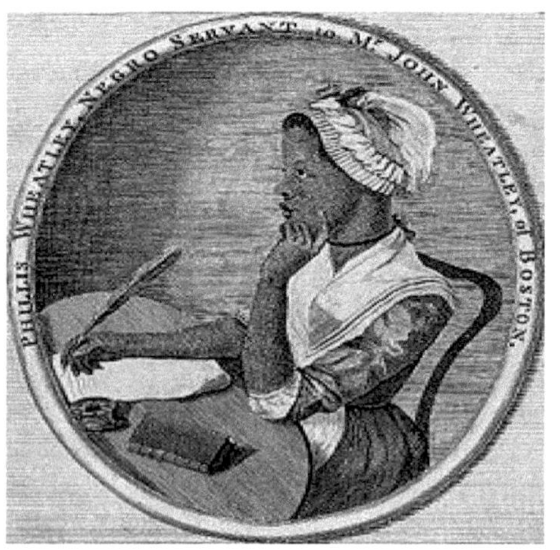

ACKNOWLEDGMENTS

I would like to acknowledge my husband Todd Walker, my parents Ophelia and Robert Jones, my children Brianna, Trinity, and Brendan Rascoe, and my in-laws Delores and Earl Washington. I would like to acknowledge Tonya and DJ Joyner for encouraging me to write this book and giving me the tools to do so. I lastly would like to thank all the people who asked me if I was pregnant. Your insensitive and nosy comments pushed me to stop being fluffy and be fit!

CONTENTS

DISCLAIMER

I am not a doctor, nutritionist, or dietician. I am also not a fitness trainer. I have no medical training at all. The information I share is based on my own experiences and information that I learned from my own research and listening to speakers.
I am a licensed Dance Educator with a Bachelor of Science degree from UNC-Greensboro. I'm licensed in Instructional Technology with a Master of Science degree from the illustrious North Carolina A&T State University. I'm also licensed in School Administration with a Master of Science degree from UNC-Chapel Hill.

The Cambridge Dictionary describes fat shaming as the act of criticizing or drawing attention to someone for being fat, making them feel embarrassed or ashamed. I, in fact, was fat-shamed by others and used that negative energy to fuel my weight loss journey. I have every right to share my thoughts, comments, and feelings about myself while on that weight loss journey. In no way, shape, or form is my book intended to fat shame or offend anyone. My only desire is that people learn to love themselves physically, mentally, emotionally and spiritually; however way they choose to manifest it in their lives.

1 UNDERWEIGHT AND STRESSED

I was 38 years old going through a separation from my now ex-husband. Let's just say I was a hot mess. The stress of the separation and impending divorce was causing me to lose my appetite. I was also working full time and in graduate school. All this while being a mother to my three spoiled darlings. So yeah, I was stressed.

It was God, family, and friends that helped me keep it together. I was slowly losing weight. My normal weight was around 116. However, when I dropped to 108, my doctor became very concerned. He stated that he thought I was underweight. He gave me some medications to improve my mood and cause me to gain weight. Boy, did I gain weight!

Soon instead of avoiding food, I turned to food

as a way to cope with my stress. I had a massive sweet tooth. Little Debbie treats were my favorite! I particularly had a love affair with honey buns. Fudge rounds were my side dude. I would literally eat a box of Little Debbie devil treats within 12 hours. I would try to hide the treats from myself by putting them in the trunk of my car. At night I would sneak into my car in the garage and grab a honey bun or two. I would even give my Little Debbie box of bakery crack to my daughter to hide from me. I would go upstairs to her room and beg for my own food! She would give in to my requests and give me one or two honey buns so that I would leave her alone.

That year I gained an extra 20 pounds so. I was now 128. I could still wear my size small clothing, but it was starting to fit a little tight. I started to notice that my belly was starting to grow and this time I wasn't pregnant.

I'm sharing my journey with you so that you might not fall prey to the sugar demon like I once did. Your demon might not be sugar. Maybe it's pasta or bread. Maybe you just overeat and binge because you are bored. Whatever the reason, let's look at ways to identify your triggers so that they no longer control you. You should be in control of your eating, not the other way around! Let's start first by creating a food diary.

I want you to write down what you eat in one

week's time. You will write down not just what you eat, but how much and when. Then I want you to seriously evaluate your eating habits. Are you eating healthy? Are you eating unhealthy? Are you a snacker? Do you binge eat? Once you know your eating habits, you can then begin to do better and eat better! Now I am not a dietitian, but I do know that this exercise will help inform you about your eating habits. To help stop emotional eating, try these tips:

1. **Keep a food diary…**Write down what you eat, how much you eat, when you eat, how you feel when you eat, and how hungry you are.

2. **Tame your stress**….I started to just walk after work. I teach my dance choreography daily and actually performing helped alleviate my stress.

3. **Have a hunger reality check….**Ok, ask yourself are you're really hungry? If you'd rather eat a Krispy Kreme donut over an apple, then you ain't really hungry.

4. **Get support….**I sought out God, friends, family, and even a therapist to get my mind, body, and spirit in check.

5. **Fight boredom....** My Daddy would always tell me to start cleaning or straighten up my home if I was bored. He always said to stay busy and stay moving!

6. **Take away temptation....**My Daddy would also say "Stay out the kitchen, Nae Nae!" Avoid it at all cost; don't give in to your nighttime cravings. Don't buy the food that triggers you to overeat!

7. **Don't deprive yourself....**Allow yourself to have a cheat meal, dessert, or a glass of wine once a week. Just not every day.

8. **Snack healthy....**Sing it with me this Blue's Clues Classic...Healthy snacks, Healthy snacks! We love to eat, YUM, healthy snacks — carrots, bananas, and celery too. We love to eat our healthy snacks.....Uh-oh!

The song speaks for itself.

Food Diary

Use this for seven days to record what you eat.

Day 1

Meal 1____

      Serving size _____   Servings_____

      Protein______   Carbs______

      Sugar______   Fat______

      Calories_____

Meal 2____

      Serving size _____   Servings_____

      Protein______   Carbs______

      Sugar______   Fat______

      Calories_____

Meal 3____

      Serving size _____   Servings_____

      Protein______   Carbs______

      Sugar______   Fat______

      Calories_____

Snack 1 ____

        Serving size _____   Servings_____

        Protein______   Carbs______

        Sugar______   Fat______

        Calories_____

Snack 2 ____

        Serving size _____   Servings_____

        Protein______   Carbs______

        Sugar______   Fat______

        Calories_____

Snack 3 ____

        Serving size _____   Servings_____

        Protein______   Carbs______

        Sugar______   Fat______

        Calories_____

Total Daily Calorie Consumption _______

Total Daily Protein Consumption _______

Total Daily Sugar Consumption _______

Total Daily Carb Consumption _______

Total Daily Fat Consumption _______

__Day 2__

Meal 1____

      Serving size _____   Servings_____

      Protein______   Carbs______

      Sugar______   Fat______

      Calories_____

Meal 2____

      Serving size _____   Servings_____

      Protein______   Carbs______

      Sugar______   Fat______

      Calories_____

Meal 3____

      Serving size _____   Servings_____

      Protein______   Carbs______

      Sugar______   Fat______

      Calories_____

Snack 1 ____

      Serving size _____   Servings_____

      Protein______   Carbs______

      Sugar______   Fat______

      Calories_____

Snack 2 _______________________________________

      Serving size _____   Servings_____

      Protein______   Carbs______

      Sugar______   Fat______

      Calories_____

Snack 3 _______________________________________

      Serving size _____   Servings_____

      Protein______   Carbs______

      Sugar______   Fat______

      Calories_____

Total Daily Calorie Consumption _______

Total Daily Protein Consumption _______

Total Daily Sugar Consumption _______

Total Daily Carb Consumption _______

Total Daily Fat Consumption _______

Day 3

Meal 1____

      Serving size ____   Servings____

      Protein_____   Carbs_____

      Sugar_____   Fat_____

      Calories____

Meal 2____

      Serving size ____   Servings____

      Protein_____   Carbs_____

      Sugar_____   Fat_____

      Calories____

Meal 3____

      Serving size ____   Servings____

      Protein_____   Carbs_____

      Sugar_____   Fat_____

      Calories____

Snack 1 _______________________________________

      Serving size ____   Servings____

      Protein_____   Carbs_____

      Sugar_____   Fat_____

      Calories____

Snack 2 ____

      Serving size _____   Servings_____

      Protein______   Carbs______

      Sugar______   Fat______

      Calories_____

Snack 3 ____

      Serving size _____   Servings_____

      Protein______   Carbs______

      Sugar______   Fat______

      Calories_____

Total Daily Calorie Consumption _______

Total Daily Protein Consumption _______

Total Daily Sugar Consumption _______

Total Daily Carb Consumption _______

Total Daily Fat Consumption _______

<u>Day 4</u>

Meal 1____

       Serving size _____   Servings_____

       Protein______   Carbs______

       Sugar______   Fat______

       Calories_____

Meal 2____

       Serving size _____   Servings_____

       Protein______   Carbs______

       Sugar______   Fat______

       Calories_____

Meal 3____

       Serving size _____   Servings_____

       Protein______   Carbs______

       Sugar______   Fat______

       Calories_____

Snack 1 ____

       Serving size _____   Servings_____

       Protein______   Carbs______

       Sugar______   Fat______

       Calories_____

Snack 2 ______________________________________

      Serving size _____   Servings_____

      Protein_____   Carbs_____

      Sugar_____   Fat_____

      Calories_____

Snack 3 ______________________________________

      Serving size _____   Servings_____

      Protein_____   Carbs_____

      Sugar_____   Fat_____

      Calories_____

Total Daily Calorie Consumption _______

Total Daily Protein Consumption _______

Total Daily Sugar Consumption _______

Total Daily Carb Consumption _______

Total Daily Fat Consumption _______

Day 5

Meal 1____

       Serving size _____   Servings_____

       Protein______   Carbs______

       Sugar______   Fat______

       Calories_____

Meal 2____

       Serving size _____   Servings_____

       Protein______   Carbs______

       Sugar______   Fat______

       Calories_____

Meal 3____

       Serving size _____   Servings_____

       Protein______   Carbs______

       Sugar______   Fat______

       Calories_____

Snack 1 ____

       Serving size _____   Servings_____

       Protein______   Carbs______

       Sugar______   Fat______

       Calories_____

Snack 2 ____

       Serving size _____   Servings_____

       Protein______   Carbs______

       Sugar______   Fat______

       Calories_____

Snack 3 ____

       Serving size _____   Servings_____

       Protein______   Carbs______

       Sugar______   Fat______

       Calories_____

Total Daily Calorie Consumption _______

Total Daily Protein Consumption _______

Total Daily Sugar Consumption _______

Total Daily Carb Consumption _______

Total Daily Fat Consumption _______

<u>Day 6</u>

Meal 1____

       Serving size _____   Servings_____

       Protein______   Carbs______

       Sugar______   Fat______

       Calories_____

Meal 2____

       Serving size _____   Servings_____

       Protein______   Carbs______

       Sugar______   Fat______

       Calories_____

Meal 3____

       Serving size _____   Servings_____

       Protein______   Carbs______

       Sugar______   Fat______

       Calories_____

Snack 1 ____

       Serving size _____   Servings_____

       Protein______   Carbs______

       Sugar______   Fat______

       Calories_____

Snack 2 ____

     Serving size _____   Servings_____

     Protein______   Carbs______

     Sugar______   Fat______

     Calories_____

Snack 3 ____

     Serving size _____   Servings_____

     Protein______   Carbs______

     Sugar______   Fat______

     Calories_____

Total Daily Calorie Consumption _______

Total Daily Protein Consumption _______

Total Daily Sugar Consumption _______

Total Daily Carb Consumption _______

Total Daily Fat Consumption _______

Day 7

Meal 1____

       Serving size _____   Servings_____

       Protein______   Carbs______

       Sugar______   Fat______

       Calories_____

Meal 2____

       Serving size _____   Servings_____

       Protein______   Carbs______

       Sugar______   Fat______

       Calories_____

Meal 3____

       Serving size _____   Servings_____

       Protein______   Carbs______

       Sugar______   Fat______

       Calories_____

Snack 1 _______________________________________

       Serving size _____   Servings_____

       Protein______   Carbs______

       Sugar______   Fat______

       Calories_____

Snack 2 ______________________________________

      Serving size _____   Servings_____

      Protein_____   Carbs_____

      Sugar_____   Fat_____

      Calories_____

Snack 3 ______________________________________

      Serving size _____   Servings_____

      Protein_____   Carbs_____

      Sugar_____   Fat_____

      Calories_____

Total Daily Calorie Consumption _______

Total Daily Protein Consumption _______

Total Daily Sugar Consumption _______

Total Daily Carb Consumption _______

Total Daily Fat Consumption _______

Another exercise I would suggest that you do is record the mood that you are in when you eat. Were you happy? Were you sad or depressed? Were you anxious or nervous? Angry? Frustrated? Were you exhausted and sleepy? Here is a 7-Day Mood Journal so that you can track your moods when you eat. At the end of the seven days, see if you have any patterns to when you eat. See how your mood may be affecting when and what you may be eating.

Day 1

Meal/Snack 1 _______________________________________

What is your mood?_____________________________________

Meal/Snack 2 _______________________________________

What is your mood? ____________________________________

Meal/Snack 3 _______________________________________

What is your mood? ____________________________________

Meal/Snack 4_______________________________________

What is your mood? ____________________________________

Meal/Snack 5_______________________________________

What is your mood? ____________________________________

Meal/Snack 6_______________________________________

What is your mood? ____________________________________

Day 2

Meal/Snack 1 _______________________________________

What is your mood?_____________________________________

Meal/Snack 2 _______________________________________

What is your mood? ____________________________________

Meal/Snack 3 _______________________________________

What is your mood? ____________________________________

Meal/Snack 4_______________________________________

What is your mood? ____________________________________

Meal/Snack 5_______________________________________

What is your mood? ____________________________________

Meal/Snack 6_______________________________________

What is your mood? ____________________________________

Day 3

Meal/Snack 1 _______________________________

What is your mood?_______________________________

Meal/Snack 2 _______________________________

What is your mood? _______________________________

Meal/Snack 3 _______________________________

What is your mood? _______________________________

Meal/Snack 4_______________________________

What is your mood? _______________________________

Meal/Snack 5_______________________________

What is your mood? _______________________________

Meal/Snack 6_______________________________

What is your mood? _______________________________

Day 4

Meal/Snack 1 _______________________________________

What is your mood?_____________________________________

Meal/Snack 2 _______________________________________

What is your mood? ____________________________________

Meal/Snack 3 _______________________________________

What is your mood? ____________________________________

Meal/Snack 4_______________________________________

What is your mood? ____________________________________

Meal/Snack 5_______________________________________

What is your mood? ____________________________________

Meal/Snack 6_______________________________________

What is your mood? ____________________________________

Day 5

Meal/Snack 1 _______________________________________

What is your mood?_______________________________________

Meal/Snack 2 _______________________________________

What is your mood? _______________________________________

Meal/Snack 3 _______________________________________

What is your mood? _______________________________________

Meal/Snack 4_______________________________________

What is your mood? _______________________________________

Meal/Snack 5_______________________________________

What is your mood? _______________________________________

Meal/Snack 6_______________________________________

What is your mood? _______________________________________

Day 6

Meal/Snack 1 ____

What is your mood?_______________________________________

Meal/Snack 2 ____

What is your mood? ______________________________________

Meal/Snack 3 ____

What is your mood? ______________________________________

Meal/Snack 4____

What is your mood? ______________________________________

Meal/Snack 5____

What is your mood? ______________________________________

Meal/Snack 6____

What is your mood? ______________________________________

Day 7

Meal/Snack 1 ___________________________________

What is your mood?___________________________________

Meal/Snack 2 ___________________________________

What is your mood? ___________________________________

Meal/Snack 3 ___________________________________

What is your mood? ___________________________________

Meal/Snack 4___________________________________

What is your mood? ___________________________________

Meal/Snack 5___________________________________

What is your mood? ___________________________________

Meal/Snack 6___________________________________

What is your mood? ___________________________________

DISCOVERY

Question #1. Take time to review your eating habits. What did you find?

____

____

____

Question #2. What did you discover about your mood when you are eating regular meals?

____

____

____

Question #3. What did you find about your mood when you eat snacks?

____

____

____

Question #4. Do you think your mood is affecting your eating habits? Why or why not?

____

____

____

DISCOVERY 2

Here is another different evaluation to see if you are an emotional eater.

Question #1. Do you munch on chips, or other salty snacks or sweets when you are bored?
     a. not very often
     b. occasionally
     c. yes, a few times a week
     d. yes, often

Question #2 Do you eat when you are stressed?
     a. Not very often
     b. Occasionally
     c. Yes, a few times a week
     d. Yes, often

Question #3 Do you reach for something to eat when you can't fix a problem that's bothering you?
     a. Not very often
     b. Occasionally
     c. Yes, a few times a week
     d. Yes, often

Question#4 Do you snack during work when you are frustrated?
     a. Not very often
     b. Occasionally
     c. Yes, a few times a week
     d. Yes, often

Question #5 How often do you have nighttime snacks when you are worried and can't sleep?

        a.   Not very often
        b.   Occasionally
        c.   Yes, a few times a week
        d.   Yes, often

Question #6 Do you tend to eat more when you are tired?

        a.   Not very often
        b.   Occasionally
        c.   Yes, a few times a week
        d.   Yes, often

Question #7 Do you tend to eat comfort foods such as mashed potatoes, macaroni and cheese, apple pie or cookies when you are at home?

        a.   Not very often
        b.   Occasionally
        c.   Yes, a few times a week
        d.   Yes, often

Question #8 What do you usually do when you are feeling lonely?

        a.   Go for a walk
        b.   Call a friend
        c.   Eat a Treat
        d.   Snack in front of the TV

If you answered all A's you typically don't eat for emotional reasons. I would suggest that you continue to set yourself up for success by having plenty of wholesome foods in your home and be prepared with healthy snacks for times when you really need it. Also, I would recommend that you continue to manage your stress and make sure to get enough rest. Hunger hormones become off balance when you have not had enough sleep. You are also more likely to snack when you are sleepy.

If you answered with mostly B's, then you sometimes eat for emotional reasons. It can be common to eat when bored or snack endlessly when you are stressed. However, I would suggest that you try to check yourself before you wreck your waistline. If you have just eaten, you are probably not physically hungry. Distract yourself by doing something to occupy your time for at least 20 minutes to give your food cravings time to subside. Fight boredom by taking a short walk, listen to your favorite music or just do another activity.

If you answer with mostly C's, then you frequently eat for emotional reasons. Put that cookie down and think about the potential consequences of your behavior. For each honey bun I consumed, I added an extra 300 calories to my diet and ultimately to my stomach, hips, thighs, and rear end. Also, think about how sluggish and tired you will feel after consuming those unnecessary calories. Stop impulsive, emotional eating by reminding yourself that this is not the best way to deal with your emotions and stress that you are going through in your life. Really think about if that food that you are about to consume is worth sacrificing your health and weight loss goals.

If you answer with mostly D's, then it appears that you seem to struggle with emotional eating most of the time. I would highly suggest that you keep a food diary to pinpoint your specific food triggers. You really need to grasp and understand your eating habits. You should also take note of your mood when you emotionally eat. Hopefully, you will see patterns that will reveal a connection between the food you eat and your feelings. A food diary will also cause you to be aware and bring to your attention the food that you have already eaten in a day. If I'd have kept a food diary when I was eating a whole box of Little Debbie's I might have realized sooner that I had consumed enough food for today and really didn't need a fourth fudge round.

Most importantly, get the support you need by talking to supportive family, friends or a therapist. Seek encouragement from them when you feel your emotional tank is almost empty. Talk to a therapist or research different strategies to deal with your emotions and stress that doesn't involve consume food.

2 HAPPY AND COMPLACENT

Well, I'm 39, and I am living my best life! I have fallen in love, child! My life is still busy and hectic. I have however made it worse by starting a part-time job while working full time. And yes, I am still in graduate school. I say all that to say this. I was NOT making time to eat healthily and exercise. My boyfriend and I would eat out at least twice a week. My babe loved to spoil me with food. After work, I would ask to go to Chili's and order my favorite meal: an Old-timers burger with black beans, fries, and sweet tea, Yum! However, this meal is an easy 1,200 in calories. Since I never missed breakfast or lunch, I unknowingly had consumed too many calories for the day.

I loved food, and I still do. Unfortunately, I ate too much of it. I was addicted to French fries, bread, pasta, and sugar. Growing up, my mom would buy wheat bread, never white. I liked to make my peanut butter and jelly sandwiches. I loved my chicken or turkey and cheese subs from subway.

My two favorite pieces of bread are from Texas Roadhouse and Red Lobster! The sweet butter biscuits from Texas Roadhouse and the cheddar cheese biscuits from Red Lobster are to die for! So yes, I was so addicted to bread.

My second favorite item that increased my weight was my addiction to coffee. Now black coffee is perfectly fine. However, I would manage to put AT LEAST 12-15 tablespoons of sugar in my eight ounces of coffee to remain awake and sane. As a teacher and grad student, I literally ran off of coffee. I would also put in two to three tablespoons of creamer or half and half in my coffee as well. So let's just say that my calorie consumption of coffee was way too high. Some days I would consume two cups of coffee a day, with the same amount of sugar and cream.

My third favorite item that increased my weight was my daily consumption of large sweet iced tea from a popular fast food establishment. I'm a southern belle who loves sweet tea. The tea was cheap no more than a dollar at some locations. Drinking that tea alone was adding an extra 250 calories to my already too much sugar-laden diet.

I know I mentioned I was happy. I still am happy. However, I was not taking the time to exercise.

I did teach dance every day in class; however, over time my body had grown used to the same amount of physical exertion. I was gaining weight because I was consuming more calories than I was burning.

I was also gaining weight because my doctor had put me on medication to stabilize my moods. A side effect of the medication was weight gain. I was also taking high blood pressure medication which was causing weight gain as well. Towards the end of the year, as I approached my 40th birthday, I had gained another ten pounds. I was now around 138.

The day before my 40th birthday, my boyfriend, (now husband) threw a spectacular 40th birthday party. No one had EVER thrown me a surprise party before! I was surprised and so grateful. My children, parents, future in-laws, friends, and his family were all in attendance. My dance team family even came and danced in my honor!

Also on that special day, my boyfriend decided to put a ring on it!. I was so surprised! I, of course, said YES! He even created a proposal video where he recorded himself asking me to marry him every day from September 16, 2015, to January 31, 2016! That video showed me how dedicated, persistent and consistent his love for me was and still is. He put so much effort into the planning of this event. I was actually looking forward to my 40s as a newly engaged woman!

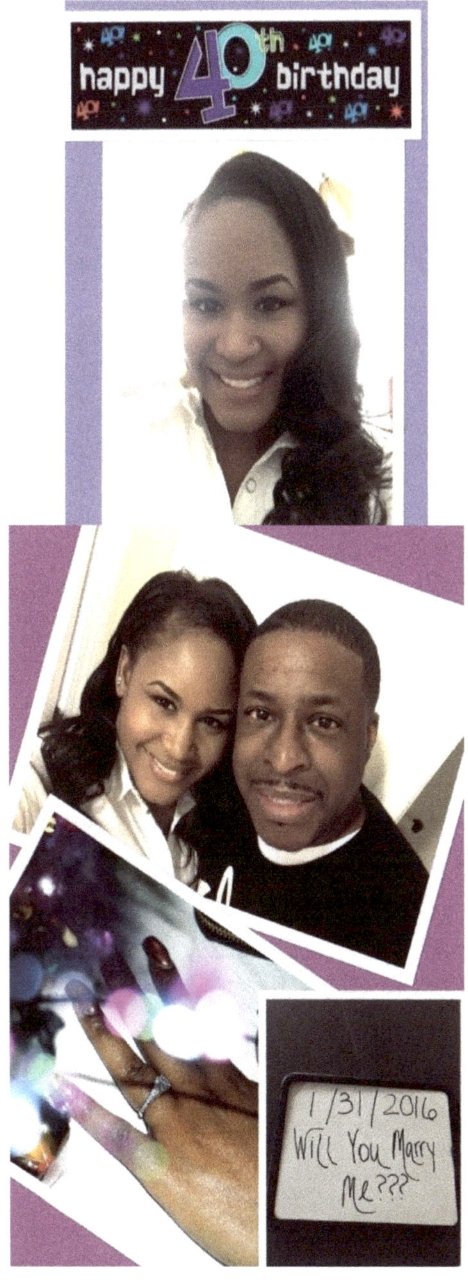
happy 40th birthday
1/31/2016
Will You Marry Me???

Chapter 2 Journal Questions:

1. List your favorite foods:

2. Are those foods listed above full of high carbohydrates?

3. Do you eat these foods when stressed?

4. Are those foods a source of comfort, yes or no?

5. Research and find some low-fat or low-carb alternatives to your above favorite foods: for example: instead of mashed potatoes try mashed cauliflower.

I'm replacing:_______________ with :_______________
I'm replacing:_______________ with :_______________
I'm replacing:_______________ with :_______________
I'm replacing:_______________ with :_______________
I'm replacing:_______________ with :_______________

3. WHO'S GOT THE JUICE!!!!

After watching the Netflix hit titled *Fat Sick and Nearly Dead* by Joe Cross. I decided I wanted to try it. I got my husband on board, and we decided to begin juicing. After shopping around, we bought a commercial grade juicer from an online retailer for a really good price. Then we started looking online for juicing recipes that would help lower high blood pressure. My mother-in-law even gave us a book of juicing recipes. I listed the ingredients for one of our favorite juices below. Your body will thank me later. You might want to stay near a bathroom because this juice is a good detox! These ingredients when juiced raw makes about 20 ounces of juice. We would take ten ounces each and drink it throughout the morning at work. I call it "The Walker Get Your Heart Right Special," and my husband calls it "The Drink of Life."

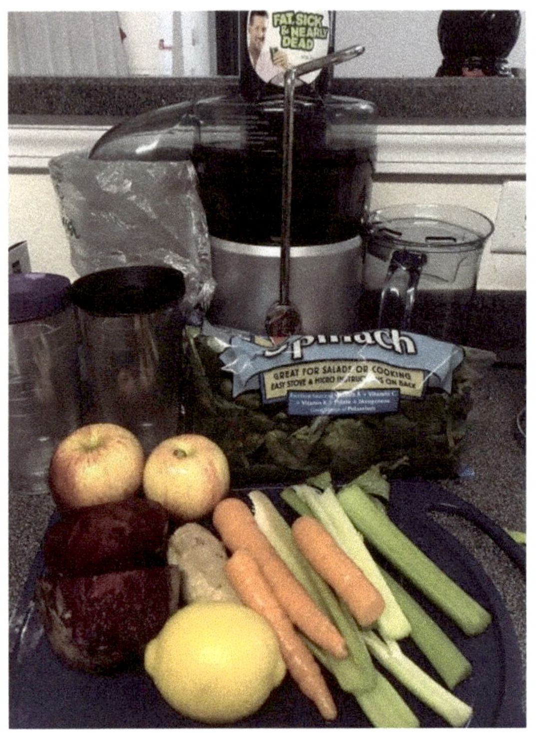

1 thumb size of a ginger root
2 Red Delicious whole apples
2 stalks of celery
2 handfuls of spinach
1 large red beet
2 medium to large sized carrots

Another favorite juice recipe I use is called 'Green Goddess Juice." This recipe makes 20 ounces of juice.

8 mandarin oranges peeled
1 whole pineapple
4 handfuls of Spinach

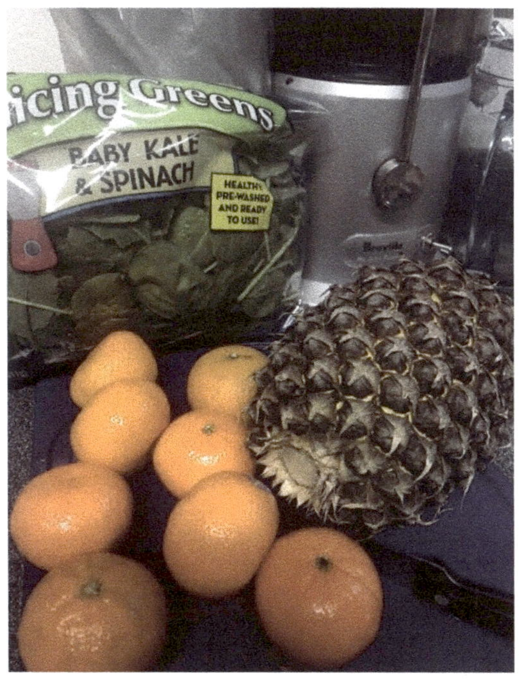

A few tips for the best results:

When using your new juicer to make these healthy, delicious and nutritious juices, make sure to follow the manufacturer's directions explicitly.

- Use organically-grown fruit and vegetables whenever possible. They are less likely to be treated with harmful pesticides and other chemicals.
- If you cannot afford organic produce, then make sure to thoroughly scrub your produce. I soak my apples in a solution of apple cider vinegar and water.
- Make sure to scrub all of your vegetables and fruits with a brush and Dawn dishwashing liquid under running water.
- I usually peel my pineapples, limes, and oranges. When I use lemons, I do not peel them. Lemon peels contain a plethora of vitamins, minerals, and fiber that can give your diet a nutritional boost.
- For leafy vegetables like spinach, parsley, collard greens, kale, lettuce, discard the outer leaves. I then would place the vegetables into a bowl a swish around so that the dirt falls to the bottom.
- Keep your produce in the refrigerator whole until use.
- To get the full benefits from the vitamins and minerals juice all fruit and vegetables raw.
- Make sure to store your juice in a sealed airtight glass container and place into the refrigerator until you are ready to enjoy the juice. I use mason jars to store my juice.

To sum it up, the Joe Cross documentary titled *Fat Sick and Nearly Dead* chronicles Joe's personal mission to regain his health. I could relate to Joe's story because I had been diagnosed with high blood pressure. I didn't want to have to take that medicine for the rest of my life. I really believed that I had high blood pressure, not because of genetics, but because I had gained an extra 30 pounds which altered my small frame. I was searching for an all-natural, healthy alternative to taking pharmaceutical drugs to lower my blood pressure.

I was also concerned about being diagnosed with type 2 diabetes by being overweight. I have a lot of relatives who have this disease. I wanted to find a natural way to help stabilize my blood sugar levels.

Please note that when I started and when I stopped taking my high blood pressure medicine I was ALWAYS under my doctor's care. I would get checkups every three months to monitor my high blood pressure. Please make sure that you see your doctor before you stop taking any medications they have prescribed for the benefit or improvement of your health!

I not only started to change my eating habits, but I realized that I needed to increase the amount of physical exercise that I was doing daily. Every time my doctor saw me he would ask about my physical activity level. I would tell him repeatedly that I taught dance for a living, so that should be enough. He would then proceed to say that I needed to do more activities that would get my heart rate up for at least thirty minutes.

So my husband and I joined a gym. I don't know about you, but it can be (and still is) hard to make it to a gym. We bought an at-home elliptical to use when we couldn't go to the gym when the weather is too cold, or raining. That elliptical stayed dormant for months, chile! I simply was not motivated enough to use it consistently. I just simply did not have the endurance to stay on that metal machinery demon more than ten minutes at a time. What I didn't realize was if that was all I could give, then that was all I could give. I simply needed to start somewhere. I knew that I needed to increase the length of time I was on the elliptical. I also needed to increase the intensity level on the elliptical over some time. I had to keep repeating to myself, "Baby steps, Nae Nae. Baby steps!"

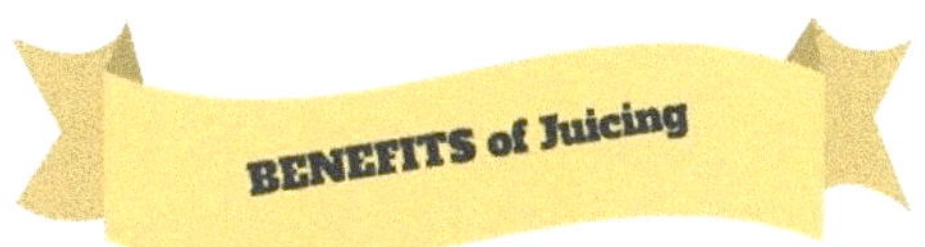

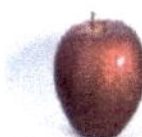

It is true an apple a day keeps the doctor away. Apples juice is not only delicious but it is rich in Vitamin C and Potassium. They are also high in fiber.

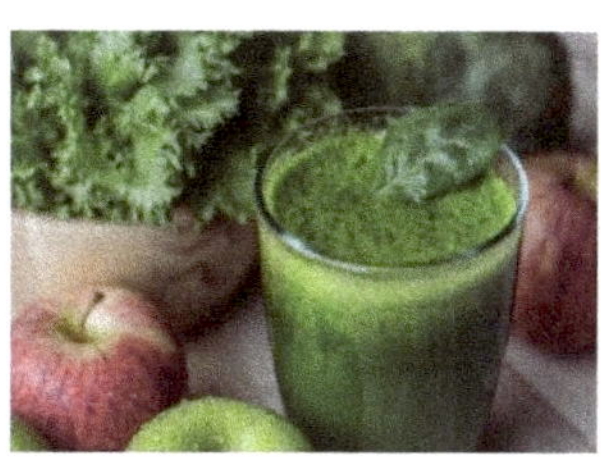

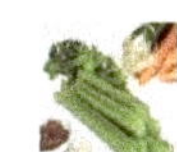

Celery juice is very high in vitamin K which promotes general bone and heart health. Fresh celery provides a source of Vitamin C, Potassium, Folate, Manganese, Calcium, Riboflavin, Magnesium, and Vitamin B6.

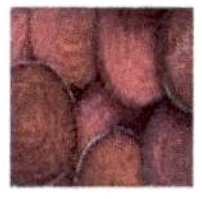

Beet juice is a good source of Folate, Vitamin C, Betaine, Manganese, Potassium Iron, Calcium, Copper and Vitamin B6. Drinking beet juice is also known to lower blood pressure considerably because of its high nitrate content.

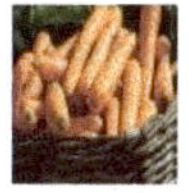

Carrots are a good source of Beta-Carotene, fiber, Vitamin K, Potassium and antioxidants. Carrots have been linked to lower cholesterol levels and improved eye health.

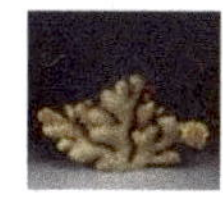

Ginger Juice does the following:
1. Anti-Inflammatory
2. Reduces Blood Pressure
3. Helps Prevent Cancer
4. Reduces Pain
5. Aids in Digestion
6. Oldest Cure for Cold
7. Lowers Cholesterol

Chapter 3 Journal Questions:

1. If you are on any prescription medicines, what are they? What steps can you take to either reduce the amount, of the frequency that you take them or eliminate them, with the guidance of a health professional?

2. What has your doctor recommended for you to do to help improve your health? For example, exercise, improve your diet.

3. Are you willing to listen to the sound advice of health professionals and make that change as Michael Jackson said in his famous song "Man in the Mirror?" I'm asking you to make that change...

4. What forms of exercise can you do now? I understand that not everyone can move around freely. However, there are forms of physical therapy that everyone can do.

5. What is the one thing that scares you the most about your current health condition? I was scared that I was going to develop diabetes and high blood pressure like so many of my relatives.

Fast forward to after my glorious wedding and phenomenal honeymoon. I'm now 41 years young, and I weighed 148 pounds. I am huge. I am fluffy. My wedding dress was a size 14! I am normally a size 2. I couldn't stand to look at myself in pictures. Below is a picture form our wedding in February 2017.

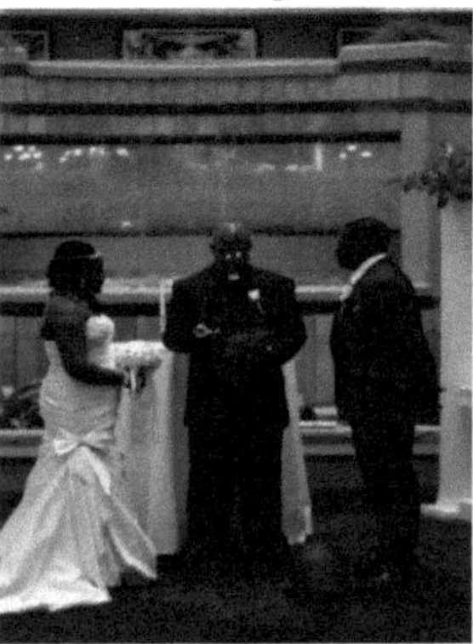

OMG, my butt and my stomach
look the same from the side!

Don't get me started on how I felt about seeing myself in my husbands' videos. SHEEESH what the hell! I honestly had been procrastinating in helping my husband edit our honeymoon and anniversary photos and videos because I didn't like the enlarged image of myself.

For this last cruise, I had to buy a whole new wardrobe. I purchased clothing that had to be loose and flowy to conceal my growing belly. My butt and thighs had grown, too. I sighed because I was upset at myself because I put on 40 pounds. My face had become round and fat. I simply did not recognize myself in the mirror. I would wear large cardigans or oversized sweaters to cover my belly. In pictures, I would even hide behind family members to hide the new me. I would wear black all the time because it was slimming. I used to love to wear color.

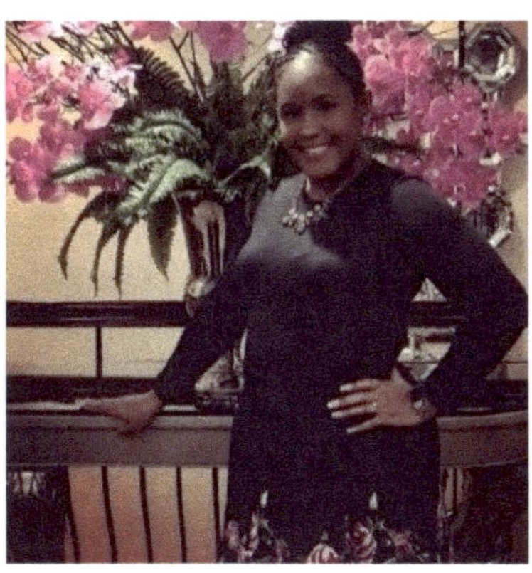

This was at my cousin's wedding the day before Thanksgiving, 2017

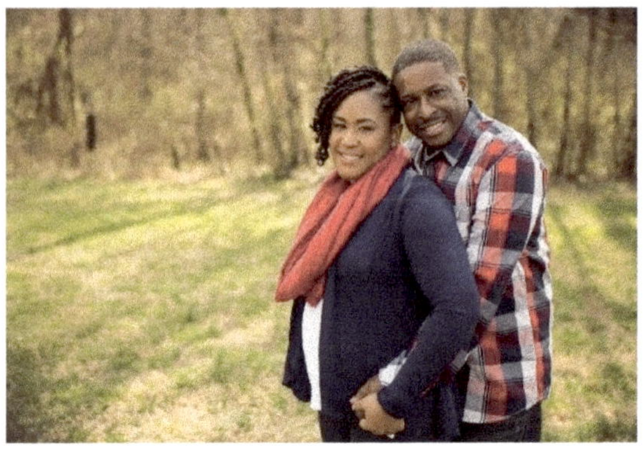

Y'all, this picture was taken in February 2018 for our anniversary photo shoot. My daughter Trinity later told me, after I had lost the 40 lbs., that this picture made her think that this was from a maternity photo shoot! She basically said I looked PREGNANT!)

To put things in perspective, when I was nine months pregnant with my children the most I ever weighted was 143. I now weighed more than when I was nine months pregnant!!!! It's sad that it took a colleague and my students to ask me on more than one occasion if I was pregnant to push me to realize that I was obese. Every time someone would ask me that rude question I would say no, I am not pregnant and give that mean stank eye. I knew however why they were asking me this question. My waist had grown to the size of when I was seven months pregnant! Fast forward to mid-2018. I knew I was over 150 pounds! That number might not mean much to you, but to me, it meant that I needed to do something fast to take control of my weight gain.

It was time to make a change in my life. I was ready to acknowledge the fact that it was time to make that change. When you are ready to make the change, you will know it.

Chapter 4 Journal Questions:

1. Have you ever been called an insensitive or rude name related to your weight? How did you respond? Did you internalize it, and get offended? Did you shrug it off and ignore it? Why?

2. As your weight has fluctuated throughout the years how has your wardrobe changed? Have you had to switch from jeans to leggings because jeans were just too uncomfortable?

3. Do you have to wear girdles, or shapewear 24-7 to keep your belly and thighs in check? How does this addition to your wardrobe make you feel?

4. If you could lose 40 pounds what would you love to be able to wear again out in public? For example, I did not feel comfortable wearing clothes that I had to tuck in because I felt that it accentuated my growing belly. A belly that I was trying to hide. I really missed wearing outfits that showed off my figure.

5 ARE YOU GOING TO BE FIT OR FAT?

Fast forward, and now I am 42 years young. I had just returned from our first-anniversary cruise. I had chaperoned the prom with the love of my life. My hairstylist for the prom told me about the gym that she attends with her fiancé. She says she has lost 20 pounds by going to the personal trainers, at this gym, who works with couples to lose weight. I decided to start going to this gym with Todd to start my weight loss journey. I also knew that I would have to dance on stage with teenagers for my annual Spring Concert. I didn't want to look like a dancing hippo on stage, so I decided to visit this local gym.

When I entered this gym on May 6, 2018, with my husband, we introduced ourselves to the gym owner and personal trainer. He proceeded to mock our outfits as soon as we walked in. The front of our outfits had the wording T & T Fitness. T & T stands for Todd and Tanae. I ordered the shirts to help motivate us to change our bodies from fat to fit. We were not fit yet, but we were on the right path to get there. My husband had bad vibes about the gym and owner from the beginning. However, we stayed for that initial 45-minute workout. The reason why my husband had bad vibes was because the gym did not properly evaluate their clients for medical history before the intensity circuit training that they were about to endure. We simply signed up online and joined the class. No one asked us if we had bad knees, heart problems, or anything that would hinder or prevent us from working out. When you go to a gym make sure that they do a proper medical evaluation before you get out there and have a heart attack!

At the end of the workout, we had a weigh in. That is when I finally had my "Ah-ha" movement. I weighed in at 158. I was thinking, *WTF??* I busted out in tears. Todd was trying to calm me down. It finally hit me that I was obese. I was fat. I just thought of myself as fluffy. At that moment something happened in my psyche. Having an excuse for not working out was not in my mindset anymore. My motivation, my focus, my passion was to get my body back in shape!

When I finally calmed down, one of the personal trainers broke down some of the measurements from the detailed weigh in. He basically said that my current muscle mass was for my 110-pound former self. My BMI, Body Mass Index, was 30.7 and my Body Fat percentage of 41.5. My Skeletal Muscle Mass was at 50.9. My BMI number, based off of my height and weight put in the category of OBESE. I had my work cut out for me, but I was willing to put in the work to lose these 40 pounds of fat!

Chapter 5 Journal Questions:

1. Have you ever experienced an embarrassing moment at a gym to where you felt judged by a personal trainer or another really fit person?

2. How did you feel after that experience? How did you cope? For example, did you turn to food, alcohol, drugs, etc?

3. After that experience did you decide to go back to that gym? Did you change gyms? Did you stop working out completely?

4. What is your ideal gym experience? Do you prefer the YMCA, Planet Fitness or doing group exercise like Zumba? Why?

5. Have you had your "Aha" moment about your weight or health? What do you think it may take for you to decide to make permanent changes to your lifestyle?

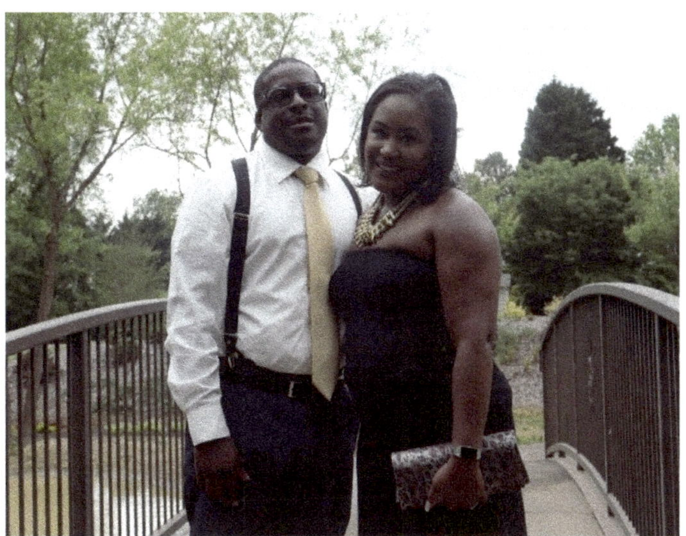

May 2018 Prom Picture, lawd have mercy, look at that belly and them ham hock arms!

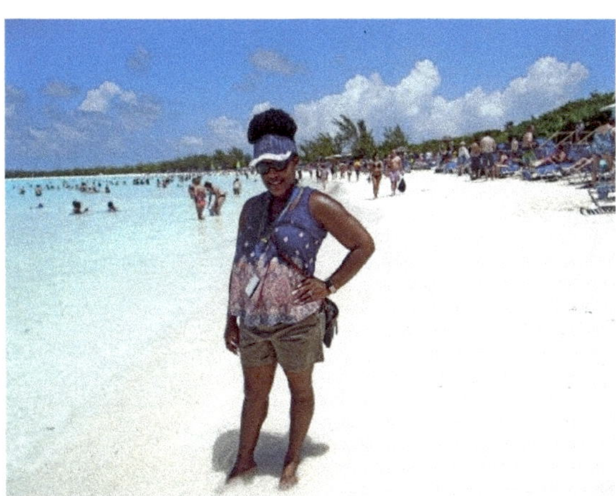

Vacationing in the Caribbean in April 2018. I didn't feel comfortable putting on a bathing suit.

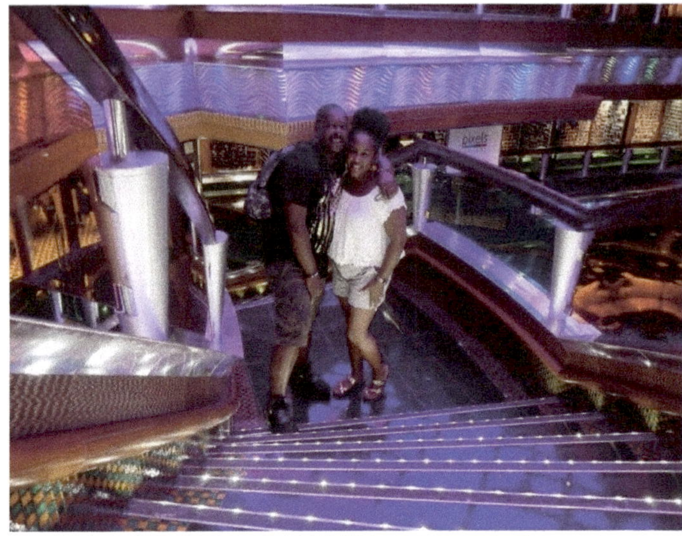

On vacation, April 2018, I'd only wear flowy tops because of my belly. The shorts I'm wearing are sz. 12.

6 GET UP AND MOVE!

So I have to admit that in the beginning, it was a STRUGGLE to get back into exercising. Like I mentioned before we started out doing intense HIIT, high-intensity interval training, workouts for 45 minutes. OMG was I sore! We went 3-4 days a week for a month to a local gym. On the days that I could not make it to the gym, I would walk for 20 minutes outside or get on my elliptical for 20 minutes. I wanted to shock my body into shape because I allowed myself to be lazy for too long. It was so hard to walk the next day the first week or two. However, after each time we went and did this intensive workout my body became more accustomed to the beating it was receiving from the trainers.

At times I wanted to quit, but I had to remember that no change will come without sacrifice. It was time to sacrifice my time, sweat, muscles aches and tears to become healthy and fit. It was time to evict my fat from my body and send it packing!

HIIT, or high-intensity interval training, workouts burn fat faster to help you slim down. Scientific researchers have even found that HIIT training for weight loss really works. HIIT is a training technique in which you give it your all, one hundred percent effort through quick, intense bursts of exercise, followed by short, recovery periods. This type of training gets and keeps your heart rate up and burns more fat in less time.

Listed below is sample Beginner HITT exercise that you can do in the privacy of your own home. You want to do these ten exercises for 40 seconds and then rest for 20 seconds. When you are resting you want to make sure that you are still moving while resting. First, start by doing a short warm-up and take some time to do some light stretches. You do not have to go in this order. You will end up working out for 10 minutes.

Squats
Push-ups
Jumping Rope
Side to Side Squats
Reverse Lunges

Side Plank
Jumping Jacks
Plank Up and Down
Knee Raises
Burpees

I've provided a sample of intermediate HITT exercises that you can do at home as well. You want to start by warming up for 5-10 minutes by jumping rope or running in place. You do not have to go in this order. You will end up working up for up to 30 minutes. You want to do each exercise for 40 seconds and then rest for 20 seconds. Repeat all ten exercised three times.

Russian Twist
Burpees
Mountain Climbers
Plank Jacks
Flutter Kicks
High Knees
Push Ups
Plank Up and Down
High Knees
Jumping Jacks

An alternative to jumping jacks is Toe-Touch Jacks.

This exercise eliminates the jumping but still uses side-to-side movement, allowing you to improve your overall balance and stability without overly stressing your knees.

How to do it: Stand tall with your feet slightly apart. Bring your arms out to the side in an X, or as high as you can comfortably go, while tapping your right foot four to six inches out to the side. Keep your weight in your left leg during the movement.

As you step your right foot back in, lower your arms back down to your sides. Repeat on the opposite side, tapping your left foot out, to complete one rep. If this is the modification for you, aim for two to three sets of eight reps.

Stair workout: I also love to utilize the stairs in my house to exercise. I run up my stairs 3-5 times then walk down. At the bottom of the stairs, I would do a series of exercises. After I did the exercises on the bottom, I would proceed to run back up the stairs 3-5 times then walk down. Listed below are the exercises I would do at the bottom of the stairs.

20 Squats
10 Push Ups
25 Crunches
25 Mountain Climbers
30-Second Plank

Chapter 6 Journal Questions

1. What was your favorite sport or physical activity that you participated in when you were growing up?

2. Do you have a favorite sport that you liked to watch live or on TV?

3. What physically hinders you from doing physical activity? (injury, illness, etc.)

4. What emotionally hinders you from doing physical activity? (anxiety, depression, etc.)

5.

    Do you have any financial reasons why you cannot afford to join a gym membership? Some organizations such as the YMCA offers programs so that people can afford the memberships. I would recommend that you ask gyms or weight loss facilities if they have such a program.

7 When Do You Eat, Sis?

I ultimately did not see any results from just going to the gym and eating relatively healthy. I also did not see significant results from drinking skinny detox teas, and detox wraps. The results from the 'teas' and 'wraps' were on temporary fixes. I was searching for a healthy lifestyle, not diet that where I would see weight loss results relatively quickly and permanently. I found that lifestyle in intermittent fasting.

Intermittent fasting is an eating style where you eat within a specific period and fast the rest of the time. Though intermittent fasting is an effective way to lose weight, it's less of a diet and more of a lifestyle choice. I stumbled onto intermittent fasting by watching YouTube videos on women who lost weight relatively quickly by doing intermittent fasting. I looked on Pinterest and discovered more information on the different types of intermittent fasting.

The following are six different intermittent fasting methods:

5:2: This method allows you to eat normally five days a week. The other two days are your fasting days, although you do still eat. Just keep it between 500 and 600 calories.

Eat-stop-eat: With this one, you restrict all food for 24 hours, once or twice a week.

16/8: You eat all of your daily calories within a shortened period — typically 6 to 8 hours — and fast for the remaining 14 to 16 hours. You can do this every day, or a few times a week. This method is also known as the Leangains protocol and was popularized by fitness expert Martin Berkhan. This method is what I do daily. I do this method of fasting by skipping breakfast and not eating anything after dinner or 8 pm.

The Warrior Diet: Fast during the day, eat a huge meal at night. The Warrior Diet was popularized by fitness expert Ori Hofmekler. Basically, you "fast" all day and "feast" at night within a 4-hour eating window. This diet proved to be the best for me in losing weight quickly.

OMAD: Another type of interment fast is called OMAD, which stands for One Meal A Day. You simply eat one large, nutritious meal in one hour. The other 23 hours you are fasting. This type of diet can be sustainable and become a lifestyle.

Switching to an intermittent fasting diet has some powerful benefits:

- **Boosts weight loss**
- **Increases energy**
- **Promotes cellular repair and autophagy (when your body consumes defective tissue to produce new parts)**
- **Reduces insulin resistance and protects against type 2 diabetes**
- **Lowers bad cholesterol**
- **Promotes longevity**
- **Protects against neurodegenerative diseases such as Alzheimer's and Parkinson's**
- **Improves memory and boosts brain function**
- **Makes cells more resilient**

Intermittent Fasting Tips: I first started to fast by just skipping breakfast. I would eat from 12-8pm. I then narrowed the window to eat from 12-5 pm or 3-8 pm. I found that you still need to count calories and need to eat healthily. If you continue to eat a high carbohydrate diet while fasting, you will increase your hunger pains, and it will be difficult to stay in the fasted state. I found that when stuck with low carb, high protein, a high vegetable diet that it was relatively easy to continue to fast through the day.

Chapter 7 Journal Questions:

1. Have you ever fasted before? What were the stipulations of the fast?

2. Why did you fast (religious, health, etc.)?

3. What diets have you tried in your lifetime? Were they successful? How long did you stay on the diet?

4. After looking at the different types of intermittent fasting which one would possibly work for you? Why?

5. Looking at the many benefits of intermittent fasting which of these benefits are you the most interested in? For example, I have relatives who have type 2 diabetes. I wanted to decrease my chances of developing this disease.

8 No, I Don't Eat Meat!

To be honest, I became a vegetarian because I didn't like how chickens and cows were treated on mega-farms and processing plants. I am well aware that not all farms are alike, which means that some farms animals are treated humanely.

I watched video footage on YouTube that showed how baby male chicks are ground alive because it is supposedly the most "instantaneous" way of killing the male chicks. Then ground up chicks go into dog food and fertilizer. The egg industry sees them as worthless because they do not lay eggs, and don't grow fast enough to be sold as meat.

I watched videos where genetically modified chickens were filled with so much growth hormone, and are too obese to even stand or even walk. I try not to consume cow milk and cheese because I saw how young dairy cows are separated from their mothers within 24 hours of birth to prevent them from nursing. The female calves will grow up to become a milk production machine just like their mothers before them. The male calves will go into the meat industry.

I am doing my part in trying to save the environment by NOT consuming meat. The production of cows, pigs, and chicken for meat is destroying our environment. I live in North Carolina, which is the 2nd top producer of pork in America. The lagoons of pork feces destroy neighbor water supplies and create air pollution. As a North Carolinian, I have driven past those rural pig farms, and the smell is disgusting. Sadly, pig farms are also normally located in poor, rural, minority areas which are also a form of environmental racism.

Hurricane Florence hit North Carolina hard, especially the pig and chicken farm industry. Dead, decomposing animals that have drowned and had laid in water for days will still be rendered and sold as the ingredients in pet food.

I did my research on how companies process meat and I determined that for my health's sake I needed to avoid all forms of processed meat at all costs. Studies show that the consumption of meat can be a factor in the cause of the following diseases and ailments:

1. **Heart Disease**- Vegetarians typically have lower cholesterol and blood pressure levels.

2. **Cancer**- Eating red meat increases your risk of cancer.

3. **Stroke**- Meat causes blockages in blood vessels which can lead to strokes.

4. **Type 2 Diabetes**- Meat is one of the most well-established dietary risks factors for diabetes.

5. **Obesity**- Everyone needs to watch how many calories they consume from meat proteins. Eating too much protein that your body does not need will turn the energy surplus of protein into fat. Eating meat contributes to obesity.

6. **Harmful Cholesterol**- The harmful cholesterol that can lead to clogged arteries and heart disease is only found in animal-based foods. A vegan diet does not contain zero cholesterol.

7. **Alzheimer's Disease**-Eating a diet rich in plant-based foods such as fruits, vegetables, and nuts help improve cognitive health.

8. **Shortened Lifespan-** Studies have shown that people who were on a vegetarian diet for more than 17 years enjoyed an increase in life

expectancy by at least 3 years.

Once I decided to become a vegetarian, I first looked for ways to substitute meals that required meat with meatless versions. In most grocery stores there are non-meat options for chicken nuggets, patties and strips. There are non-meat versions of beef such as veggie patties, beef strips, and ground beef. When I cook spaghetti, I substitute ground turkey for meatless grounds. In my salads, I add meatless chicken strips for some added protein.

Now if you're one who can't stand the taste of meatless substitutes, then there are plenty of vegetables, legumes, and grains that will give you the protein that you need in your diet. Below is a list of 20 non-dairy vegetarian sources of protein:

1. Oatmeal
Oats are a very versatile grain. You can grind it down into flour; you can use it as a binding agent in cookies and other recipes. It's a great meal for breakfast.
26 grams of protein per cup

2. Beans
Black beans, white beans, kidney beans provide you not only protein but are rich in fiber and vitamins. Beans can be used as a meat substitute, in baked goods, soups, loaves of bread, and even mixed into a salad.
39-65 grams of protein per cup (depending on variety)

3. Broccoli

Now truthfully, you would have to consume a great deal to get a significant amount of protein. The benefits of this vegetable are that it is a low-calorie food that you can snack on throughout the day for a boost in your daily protein. Broccoli is also high in Vitamin C and Vitamin A, Vitamin B6, magnesium, iron, and calcium. It can be sautéed, roasted, steamed, raw, or blended into a soup–it has a plethora of options.

17 grams of protein per bunch

4. Nut Butters

I love peanut butter. However, it has to be in moderation. Nut butters are a fantastic protein source, however they're also rich in fats and calories. A commonly known nut butter is peanut butter, but many opt for the almond version or even cashew. You could try opting for a natural source to keep it clean and sugar-free.

8 grams of protein per 2 tbsp. (Depending on the variety)

5. Spinach

Spinach is a food I hated growing up. I used to watch Popeye eat and think that it was so disgusting. Now as an adult, I realize that there was a reason my mother was always putting it on your plate. Spinach is superfood! Spinach is so versatile due to its mild flavor. It is perfect as a salad base, on a sandwich, mixed into a smoothie (you can't taste it!), juiced or steamed/sautéed for a delicious experience.

8 grams of protein per 10 oz. package

6. Tofu

Tofu is a food that I can only eat when it's cooked correctly. It is spongy and absorbs the flavor of the marinade you choose. I like when my tutu it's firm, not mushy. Tofu is a curd that is made from soybeans and pressed into blocks. Often used in Asian cuisine, it's grown wildly popular as a staple protein for many on a vegan or plant-based diet. There are so many ways to create with it.

20 grams of protein per cup

7. Quinoa

I was first introduced to Quinoa ("keen-wah") when I order a salad from Panera Bread. I now love to add this grain to my salads for an added boost of protein. The seed called quinoa can replace pasta and rice. This is not a grain. Since it's versatile and can be used on hot or cold recipes, it's no wonder it's made a name for itself as a great health food.

8 grams of protein per cup, cooked

8. Lentils

Lentils are versatile, mild, easy to cook, and rich in vitamins like iron. Lentils are often used in Indian cuisine. They are also a great substitute for meat for tacos.

18 grams of protein per cup

9. Flax Seeds

Flax seeds have a really subtle flavor to them, which makes them great for mixing into foods to get that extra fiber and protein without needing to sacrifice taste to get the benefits. I sprinkle a tablespoon of flax seeds on my daily salad. Whether you use ground flax or whole, they are really easy to blend into smoothies and mix into bread dough.

31 grams of protein per cup, whole

10. Non-Dairy Milk

There are several types of dairy-free kinds of milk now. From soy, almond, coconut, cashew & even oat, there are amazing alternatives that shockingly even contain protein because of the plant-based foods they're derived from. I use almond milk in my smoothies and in my cereal. The amount of protein it offers is small, but it is worth mentioning.

2-4 grams per 8 oz. serving, depending on the variety.

11. Nuts

Nuts are a great snack for when you are on the go and you need a little boost of protein. Walnuts, almonds, peanuts, cashews, pistachios all bring in a good serving of protein. They also, however, bring in a good serving of fats and calories too, so enjoy them in moderation.

27 grams of protein per cup, mixed nuts (roasted)

12. Avocado

Avocados are versatile as a spread, a dip, on avocado

toast, used in recipes to replace fats (like butter) or enjoyed as-is with a spoon and some seasoning. I love sliced avocados on my vegetable omelets.

4 grams of protein per average avocado

13. Split Pea

I really hated eating cooked peas as well as a child. Pea protein is beginning to be used more in vegan food and protein powders because many who adhere to a vegan diet also are careful to not consume too much soy. Pea protein can be used to make soup. It's also a common ingredient in vegetarian and vegan Indian cuisine!

16 grams of protein per cup

14. Soybeans

Soybeans are used to make tofu and tempeh. Soybeans can be snack food when you roast and salt them.

37 grams of protein per cup (dry roasted)

15. Tempeh

Tempeh is the more flavorful alternative to tofu. It's got an entirely different texture and earthier, nuttier taste to it. You can marinate and cook it just like you would tofu. Tempeh comes in a small loaf, but it's actually packed soybeans that have been cooked and fermented before taking this loaf-like shape you see in the store.

31 grams of protein per cup

16. Vegan Protein Powder

The vast majority of protein powders use whey protein

which is derived from cow's milk. Vegan protein powder is now on the market today are used a great deal by vegan athletes. Many protein powders use pea protein or soy. I use the vegan protein powder called Vega Protein & Greens with pea protein in my smoothies. It gives me 20g of protein per serving.

17. Meat Substitutes

I personally use the following meatless brands in my meals: Quorn, Morning Star, and Gardein. I can feel comfortable knowing that my meals don't lack protein even though they're meat-free. Often brands such as these make meat substitutes that are made from pea or soy proteins. Each brand has varying nutritional labels, which is why it's always important to read your labels and consider which have the best nutritional qualities for your diet!

18. Chia Seeds

I add a tablespoonful of Chia seeds to my smoothies to help curb my hunger and help me feel fuller longer. They have the ability to take on liquid and grow over double their size into gelatinous balls. Since it turns gelatinous, it's even able to be used as a pudding base when combined with dairy-free milk!
4 grams of protein per tablespoon

19. Nutritional Yeast

Vegans are obsessed with it because it helps give foods a taste similar to cheese. Being a former heavy cheese connoisseur, I can attest it does not taste like cheese. It is easy to cook with or sprinkle on your salads and meals for a parmesan cheese-like experience. It's rich in B Vitamins, but also very high in protein considering its calories.

9 grams of protein for 2 tablespoons

20. Hemp Seeds

Hemp Seeds are a complete protein. These tiny seeds are easy to add to any meal. It contains a sizable amount of magnesium, iron, calcium, zinc, and selenium. It is also a good source of omega-3 and omega-6 fatty acids. Interestingly, some studies indicate that the type of fats found in hemp seed may help reduce inflammation, as well as diminish symptoms of PMS, menopause and certain skin disease.

13 grams of protein in 3 tablespoons

Chapter 8 Journal Questions:

1. What are your favorite vegetables?

2. How often and how many vegetables do you eat daily?

3. Have you ever tried a veggie burger? Would you be willing to try one made at home or at a restaurant? Why?

4. What was your relationship with vegetables growing up? Did you love them? Hate them? Why?

5. If you could give up eating poultry, beef or pork which would it be? Why?

6. Which meat would be the hardest to give up? Why?

9 Ok, I Eat Fish Now!

A pescetarian, by definition, is someone who chooses to eat a vegetarian diet, but who also eats fish and other seafood. It's a largely plant-based diet of whole grains, nuts, legumes, produce and healthy fats, with seafood playing a key role as the main protein source. Many pescatarians also eat dairy and eggs.

I became a pescetarian for a few reasons. One, I was getting bored eating the same familiar vegetarian foods. Secondly, it is extremely hard to eat out and eat vegetarian. I didn't want to always have just a salad when I'm eating at a restaurant. Thirdly, my father-in-law makes the best fried whiting on the planet. He and his wife Delores use to own a seafood restaurant named East Market Seafood located in Greensboro, North Carolina. One day I came by his home, and he was frying up his fish. I gave into temptation and had a serving or two.

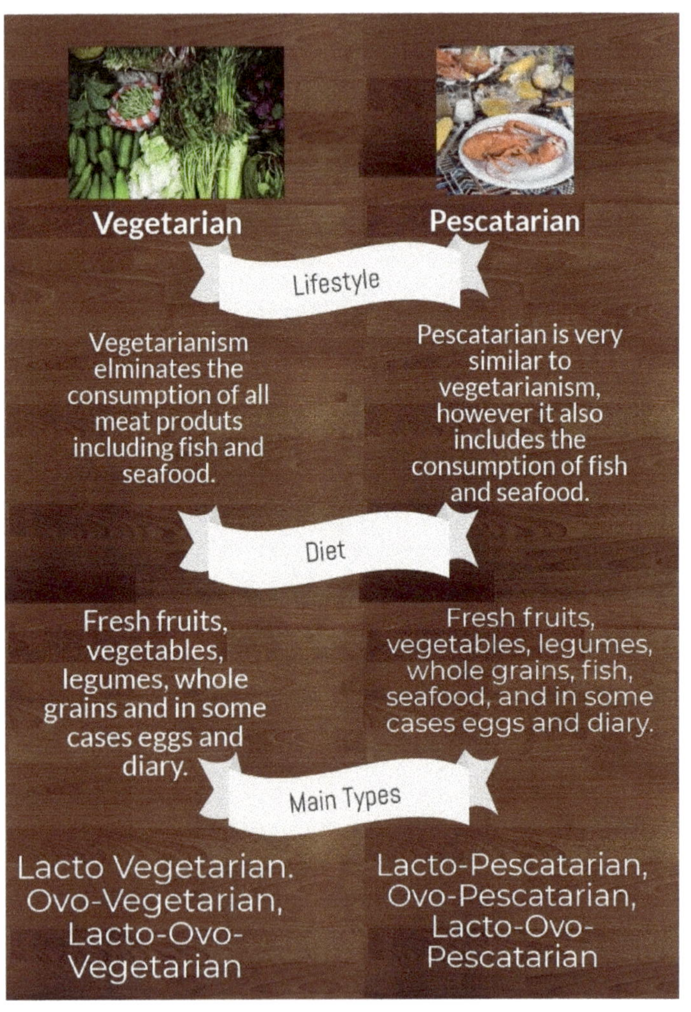

Vegetarian
Pescatarian
Lifestyle
Vegetarianism elminates the consumption of all meat produts including fish and seafood.
Pescatarian is very similar to vegetarianism, however it also includes the consumption of fish and seafood.
Diet
Fresh fruits, vegetables, legumes, whole grains and in some cases eggs and diary.
Fresh fruits, vegetables, legumes, whole grains, fish, seafood, and in some cases eggs and diary.
Main Types
Lacto Vegetarian. Ovo-Vegetarian, Lacto-Ovo-Vegetarian
Lacto-Pescatarian, Ovo-Pescatarian, Lacto-Ovo-Pescatarian

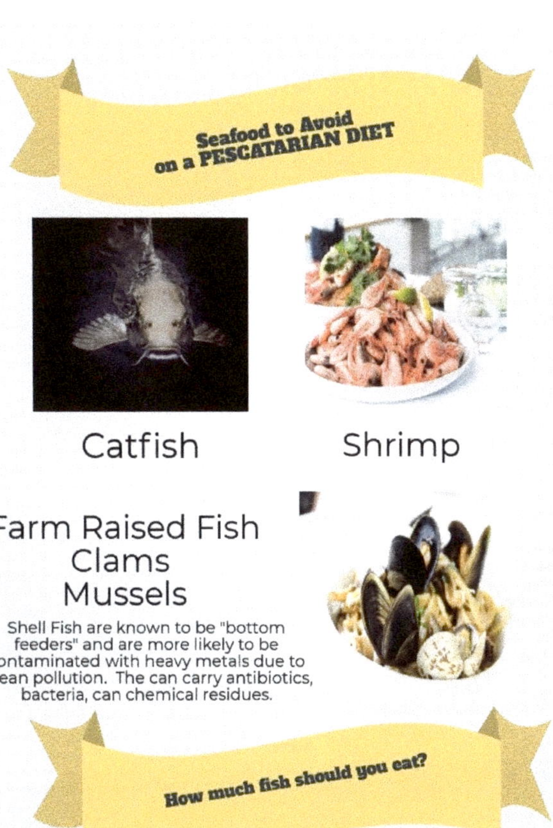

Some experts
recommend eating fish
at least 2-3 times a
week.

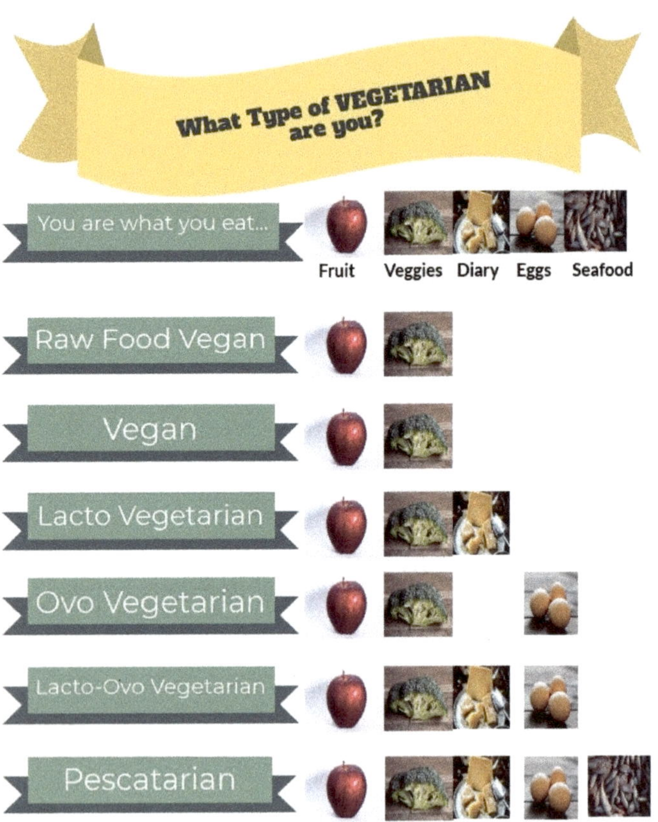
What Type of VEGETARIAN are you?
You are what you eat...
Fruit   Veggies   Diary   Eggs   Seafood
Raw Food Vegan
Vegan
Lacto Vegetarian
Ovo Vegetarian
Lacto-Ovo Vegetarian
Pescatarian

Chapter 9 Journal Questions

1. Growing up which was your favorite seafood meal?

2. Has your favorite seafood changed since you are older?

3. If one of your favorite seafood meals is on the not recommend list will you stop eating it? Why?

4. Why do you think you should not eat seafood daily?

5. Which of the several health benefits of eating seafood listed above are you the most interested in? Why?

10 VEGETARIAN VS. VEGAN WHAT IS THE DIFFERENCE?

My decision to become a vegetarian initially was
strictly for health reasons only. I wanted to stop the
generational curse of obesity, type 2 diabetes, and high
blood pressure that plagued my family. I researched
how the life expectancy of people who ate a plant-based
diet lived longer than meat eaters. I also watched
documentaries on slaughterhouses which then made me
not want to consume food that was made from animals
for an animal rights issue. I also see that eating meat is
causing an environmental crisis worldwide. The grain
that is being used to feed the animals that are killed for
food would end world hunger. If you don't believe me
look it up. The difference between vegetarian and
vegans is that vegetarians don't eat any animals,
including pigs, chickens, cows, fish, and all others.
Vegans are more extreme and do not consume any

animal flesh, dairy, or any other product derived from an animal. I will be honest with you. I love honey and vegans do not consume honey because it comes from bees.

The main reason why I do not consider myself a 'vegan' is because to become a vegan it is a lifestyle and not a diet. The Vegan Societies definition of veganism is as follows: Veganism is a way of living which seeks to exclude, as far as is possible and practicable, all forms of exploitation of, and cruelty to, animals for food, clothing or any other purpose.

In short, the vegan lifestyle is not just about not eating food that doesn't have any animal by-products. Veganism is about not wearing animals such as fur, wool, leather, or silk because to wear these items promotes the harm and death of animals.

Vegans also only use makeup and skin care products that are not tested on animals or vegan. Many people don't know that some lipsticks and other cosmetics use to contain spermaceti from the sperm whale which was typically the type of wax used for cosmetics. Countries around the world later placed a moratorium on whaling, so cosmetics companies were forced to completely replace whale oil in lipstick and other cosmetics. Cosmetic companies replaced whale oil with beeswax and plant-based jojoba oil. Nowadays I make an effort to only buy cruelty-free or vegan makeup and cosmetics for my skin care needs.

One day I may replace my favorite wool coat with an alternative nonanimal by-product clothing item. I collect used Michael Kors purses that are made of leather. I do not plan on not wearing them or not buying any more purses. I have a couple of Anne Klein professional heels and leather boots that I also do not plan on getting rid of as well.

Another reason I have not completely converted to veganism is the fact that there are almost zero vegan restaurants in my area. One day I would love to buy a restaurant and sell vegan food; however, I am not yet in a position to do so at this time. As a vegetarian, I rarely eat out because it is so hard to find vegetarian food that is not just limited to the salad. Sometimes I have to eat a cheese pizza or pasta with Alfredo sauce with no meat so that I can order something when I do go out. Another vegan menu item of choice is French fries. Let me just tell you what I am sick and tired of French fries and salads! Most of my meals are prepared at home anyway to save money and so that I can eat.

My reasons for not committing to the lifestyle of veganism is pretty vain. I, however, can say that my actions of not eating meat and being a vegetarian are helping the environment, saving animals and has definitely improved my health and wellbeing.

11 MY FAVORITE VEGETARIAN RECIPES

It was extremely hard to narrow my favorite recipes down to 7! Don't worry one of my next books will be a cookbook with illustrations that will list all of my favorite Vegetarian and Vegan Dishes! Here are my top 7 go to Healthy Dishes.

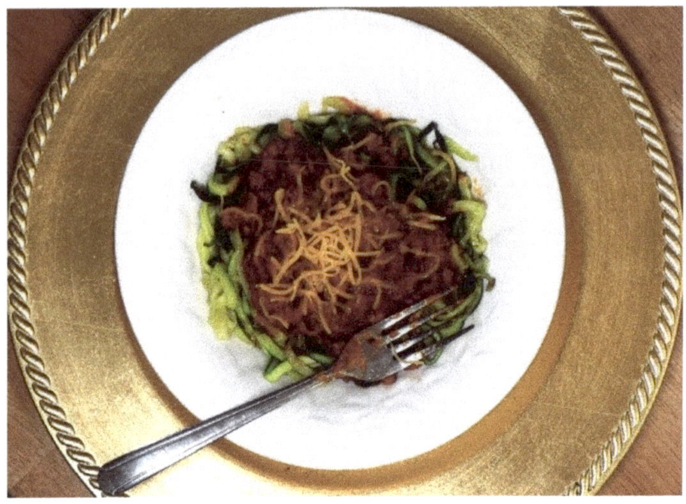

Zucchini Spaghetti

Ingredients:

- 1-2 zucchini
- Spiralizer
- Quorn meatless crumbles
- Spaghetti sauce of your choice 12-16 oz.
- 1 tablespoon of olive oil
- salt or sea salt
- garlic powder

Directions:

1. Warm up the spaghetti sauce on low to medium in a saucepan. Add the meatless crumbles to the spaghetti sauce.

2. You can also purchase zucchini noodles already sliced in the grocery store if you don't want to purchase a spiralizer. You can also use a

zucchini spiralizer to create your zucchini spirals into a small bowl. There is no need to peel your the zucchini skin provides extra nutrients and dietary fiber. After you spiralize your noodle cover them with a paper towel and allow the towel to soak up the excess water from the noodles for 10 minutes.

3. Transfer those zucchini spirals to a pan to sauté with the olive oil. Add the salt and garlic powder to the noodles for seasoning.

4. You only need to cook the noodles 2-3 minutes. Another cooking method is that you could also boil your zucchini noodles instead for a minute. However, whichever method you choose DO NOT overcook the noodles, or they will become soggy and taste gross!

5. Combine your zucchini noodles and sauce however you desire and bon appetit!

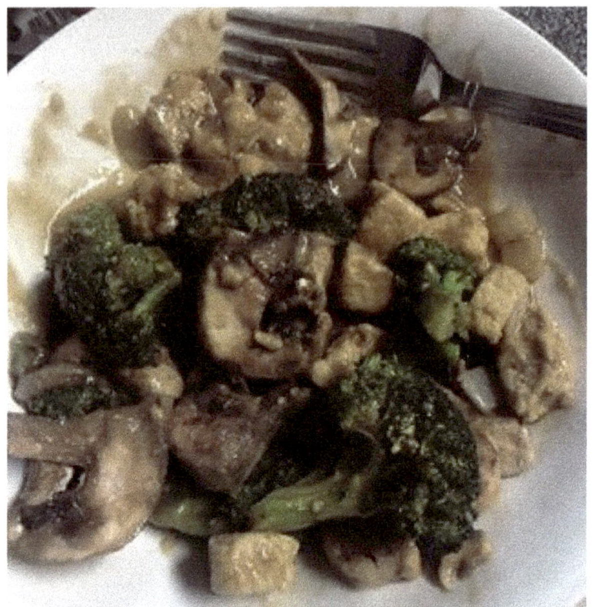

**Chinese Broccoli, Mushroom with
Meatless Chicken in Garlic Sauce**

Indigents:
- 1 onion (diced)
- 4 cloves garlic (minced)
- 3 tablespoons olive oil
- 2 cups broccoli (chopped)
- 8 oz. of mushrooms
- 1 package of Quorn Meatless Chicken pieces
- 1 ½ teaspoon ginger powder
- 1/4 teaspoon cayenne pepper
- ¼ cup of flour
- ¼ cup of honey
- ¼ cup of soy sauce

- 1 cup of vegetable stock
- 2 tablespoons Sesame oil

Directions:

1. Chop the broccoli, chop up the mushrooms, dice the onion, and mince the garlic.
2. In a large skillet, sauté onions, mushrooms, minced garlic and in olive oil until the onions turn clear, about 3 to 5 minutes.
3. Add the meatless chicken pieces, cayenne, and broccoli to the pan and continue to cook until broccoli is done, another 6 to 8 minutes.
4. In a separate small bowl, mix together the flour, soy sauce, sesame oil, honey, ginger powder, and vegetable stock, then add this mixture to the broccoli and meatless chicken pieces.
5. Cook until sauce thickens, then remove from heat.
6. Serve the broccoli and meatless chicken pieces in garlic sauce over rice.

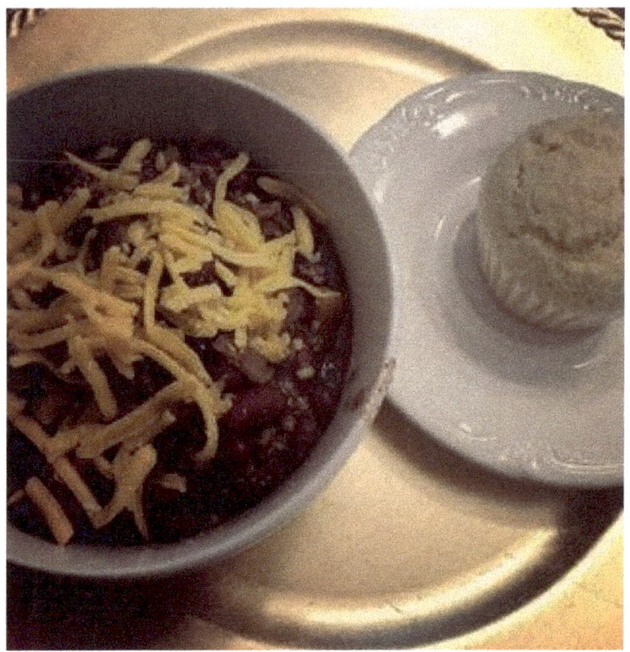

The Ultimate High Protein
Vegetarian Chili

Ingredients:
- 1 package meatless crumbles
- 1 tablespoon minced garlic
- One 16-oz can of diced tomatoes
- 2 tablespoons chili powder
- 1 teaspoon ground cumin
- 1 teaspoon ground oregano
- 1 teaspoon salt
- 1 teaspoon of black pepper
- 1/4 teaspoon cayenne pepper
- 1 cup of quinoa

- 1 medium sized diced yellow or white onion
- One 15-ounce can kidney beans, drained and rinsed
- One 15-ounce can black beans, drained and rinsed
- 1 tablespoon of olive oil
- Shredded Cheddar, for serving

Directions:

1. In a medium saucepan, combine the quinoa and water. Cook over medium heat until water is absorbed, about 15 minutes. Set aside.
2. In a large pot, heat the olive oil over high heat. Add the onion and cook until tender, about 5 minutes.
3. Add the black beans, kidney beans, tomatoes, and minced garlic.
4. Stir in the cooked quinoa.
5. Season with chili powder, oregano, cayenne pepper, cumin, salt, and black pepper. Simmer chili on low for about 30 minutes. Serve warm

I love this comfort meal! I serve this meal with my favorite side, vegetarian Jiffy cornbread. When I make my Jiffy cornbread I substitute the egg for applesauce. I also substitute the cow's milk with almond milk. You will not taste a difference!

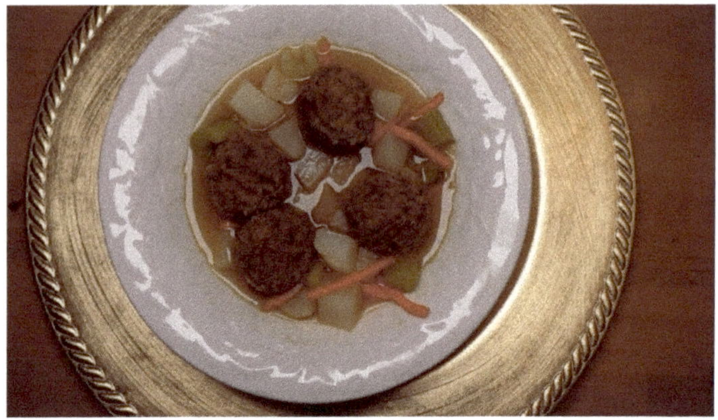

Italian Meatless Meatball Soup
(Disclaimer: In the picture about I did not add tomatoes because my husband dislikes tomatoes in his soup.)

Ingredients:

- ¼ cup parmesan cheese, grated
- 1 tablespoon extra-virgin olive oil
- 1 onion, diced
- 3 medium carrots, diced
- 3 stalks of celery, diced
- 2 cups potatoes, diced
- 3 cloves garlic, minced
- 6 cups beef or vegetable broth
- One 15 ounce can of fire roasted tomatoes, undrained
- 1 teaspoon Italian seasoning
- 2 bay leaves
- 1 teaspoon Worcestershire sauce

- salt and pepper
- parmesan cheese for serving, if desired
- 1 bag meatless meatballs by Quorn, Gardein or of Morningstar Farms
- basil for serving, if desired

Directions:

1. Heat oil in a large pot.
2. Add meatballs making sure not to overcrowd the pan. (You may have to do two batches).
3. Cook on medium high heat for 3-4 minutes on each side.
4. Take meatballs out of the pan.
5. Add in more oil if needed. Add in onion, carrots, celery, and potatoes. Sauté for 3-4 minutes.
6. Add in garlic and cook for an additional minute.
7. Stir in broth, tomatoes, seasoning, bay leaves and Worcestershire sauce.
8. Bring to a boil then simmer for 30 minutes.
9. Add meatballs back to the soup and cook until the meatballs are cooked all the way through and the potatoes are tender.
10. Season with salt and pepper to taste.
11. Serve hot with parmesan cheese and basil if desired.

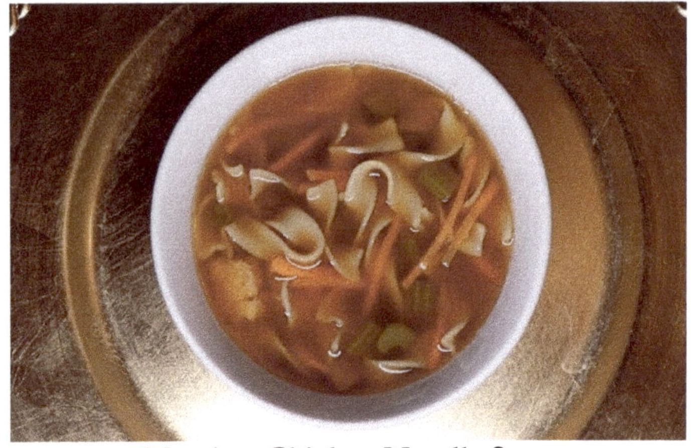

Meatless Chicken Noodle Soup

This winter has been brutal when it comes to sickness. The flu bug and a very bad cold virus swept through my school like wildfire. My husband and I ended up succumbing to the cold virus that had us out for two weeks. I managed to make a batch of meatless chicken noodle soup that helped us recovery quicker.

Ingredients:

- 2 tbsp. extra-virgin olive oil
- 1 medium onion, chopped
- 2 tablespoons of minced garlic
- 1 cup of shredded carrots
- 2-3 celery ribs, sliced
- 1 package of Quorn meatless chicken pieces
- 6 cups vegetable or chicken broth
- 12 oz. dried wide egg noodle
- salt and pepper to taste

Directions:

1. Heat oil in a large Dutch oven over medium heat. Add onions, garlic, carrots, and celery.
2. Cook and stir for 3 minutes; add the meatless chicken pieces.
3. Cook for an additional 5 minutes or until vegetables are softened, but not browned.
4. Add broth and bring to a boil. Once the mixture is boiling, add egg noodles and simmer for 8 minutes.
5. The noodles will be slightly undercooked, but don't worry–they'll continue cooking after removed from heat. This way, the noodles won't be mushy.
6. Season with salt and pepper before serving.

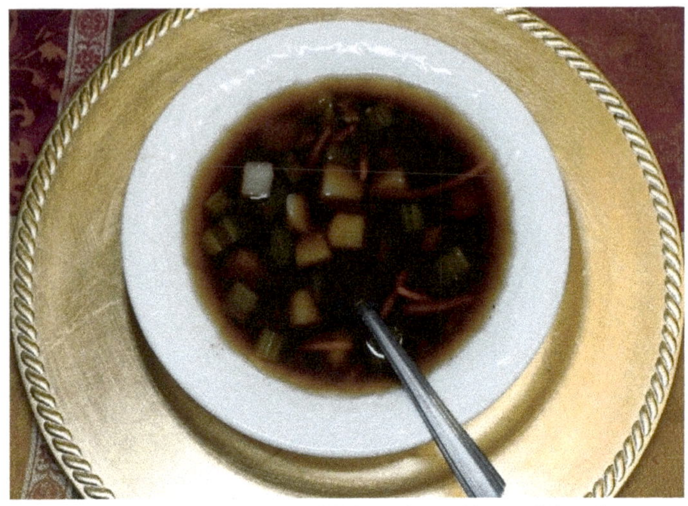

Vegetarian Potato and Meatless Crumbles Soup

This recipe is my husband's favorite soup. Once we went vegetarian, I modified it by using vegetarian stock instead of chicken stock. I also use nutritional yeast and vegan cheese instead of dairy cheese. Listed below is my recipe.

Ingredients:

- 1 bag of diced potatoes with onions
- 1 tablespoon of garlic
- 1 cup of shredded carrots
- 2 stalks of celery chopped
- Half a bag of meatless crumbles
- Salt and pepper to taste
- Nutritional yeast to taste
- Vegan or vegetarian shredded cheese (go veggie brand is what is use)

- 6-8 cups of vegetarian broth

Directions:
1. Add the vegetable broth, meatless crumbles, the bag of the potatoes and onions, garlic and season with salt and pepper. Bring to a boil, and then reduce to a slow simmer.
2. Add in the chopped celery and shredded carrots. Cover and allow to cook, stirring occasionally, for 20 to 25 minutes, or until the potatoes are soft.
3. Taste and season lightly with salt, pepper, and nutritional yeast.
4. Garnish with your choice of dairy: cheddar cheese or Vegan Cheese Shreds.

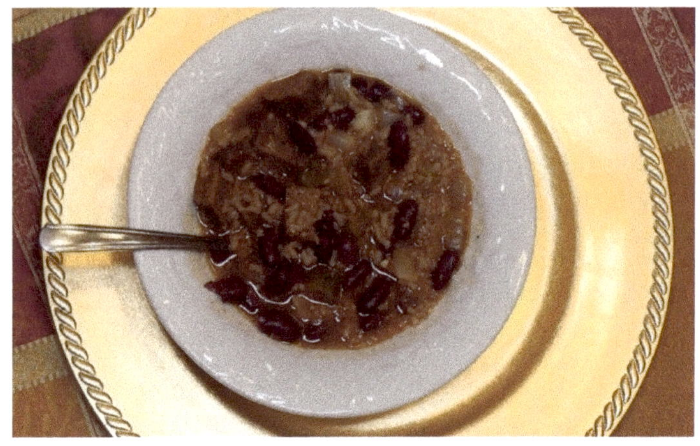

Louisiana Red Beans, Sausage and Rice

I was inspired to cook this recipe after seeing a post of a picture of this meal on Instagram. In this recipe, you can add green peppers, but I am not because I am not a peppers fan. When I make this recipe, it is only for one person, me myself and I since I am the only one who likes Cajun food. This recipe yields 3-4 servings. I would recommend that if you are making this for your family or want more leftovers, then I would double the entire recipe.

Ingredients:
- 2 tablespoon of olive oil
- 2 tofurky Italian sausages
- 1 onion, diced
- 1 rib of celery
- 2 tablespoons of minced garlic
- 2 cups of vegetable broth

- 1 can of red kidney beans, drained and rinsed
- 1 cup of brown rice
- creole seasoning

Directions:

1. Add olive oil to a Dutch oven over medium heat. Add in the sliced onion, and celery. Cook for 7-8 minutes until the onions are translucent.
2. Add in the garlic and cook for a minute.
3. Add the broth and bring to a boil over medium heat.
4. Add in the sausage, beans, and rice.
5. Add in creole seasoning and allow for the brown rice to cook for 12-15 minutes.
6. Cook until the rice is tender.

12 YOUR GUT & OVERALL HEALTH

When I was going through my separation to my now ex-husband, I was depressed, and I suffered from anxiety. My diet was also very poor. A few years have since passed, and my husband has noticed that my mood has improved along with my anxiety since becoming vegetarian. I am not saying that if you become a vegetarian or vegan that you no longer will have to take antidepressant and anxiety medication. Depression and anxiety can range from mild to severe. However, I am saying that eating a more plant-based vegetarian diet has improved my mental health.

Hippocrates is quoted to have said that "All disease starts in the gut". As a society, we have not learned that the digestive system and the brain are connected. Our gut is our second brain. I need to give y'all a science lesson so just bear with me.

The reason why you get 'butterflies" in your stomach when you become anxious is because your brain and stomach are linked. The gut contains what is called the Vagus nerve, the longest of 12 cranial nerves. This nerve runs outside the brain and through the digestive system controlling digestion and our heart rate. It is the primary channel between millions of nerve cells in our intestinal nervous system and our central nervous system, which comprises the brain and spinal cord.

Everyone knows that there are good and bad bacteria in our gut. The bacteria in our gut directly affect the function of the cells along the Vagus nerve. And some of the gut's nerve cells and microbes release neurotransmitters that speak to the brain in its own language.

The neurons in our stomach are so massive that scientists are calling the stomach the second brain! This second brain not only regulates muscle function, immune cells, and hormones but also manufactures an estimated 80 to 90 percent of serotonin! Yes, even Serotonin!

Serotonin is a neurotransmitter. It is present in our bodies mainly in the gastrointestinal tract, blood platelets, and central nervous system. Scientists believe that Serotonin is believed to regulate mood, intestinal activity and appetite, memory, and sleep.

There are two other factors that affect gut health they are GABA and Glutamate. GABA is an amino acid produced by gut bacteria that calms nerve activity by inhibiting transmissions and normalizing brain waves, helping return the nervous system to a steadier state after it's been excited by stress. Glutamate is a neurotransmitter that is produced by gut bacteria. It is involved in cognition, learning, and memory. Glutamate is abundant in a healthy brain. Scientists link a plethora of neurological issues — including anxiety, behavioral issues, depression, and Alzheimer's — have been attributed to a lack of GABA and Glutamate.

When I was seeking therapy when I was feeling low and suffered from anxiety, my therapists did not discuss my diet and how it could affect my mental health. Maybe they were not aware, or they wanted to just prescribe medication. Whatever the case may be, I have learned that there are many neurologists and psychiatrists that are now realizing that dietary changes can be more effective than antidepressants in some cases.

I by no means want to say that depression and anxiety can be eliminated solely through diet. Mental health issues are complex by nature and vary in severity. I am suggesting that improving your diet will improve your mental clarity and well-being.

So do you see now that the health of your gut

affects not only your physical health but your mental health as well?

Here is a list of foods to limit in your daily diet order to improve the health of your gut: processed foods, gluten, dairy, sugar, artificial sweeteners, caffeine and casein proteins which are found in dairy.

Here is a list of foods to improve your mood. That rhymes hehehe!

1. Dark Leafy Greens: A Nutrient-Dense Inflammation Fighter

Spinach, kale, and Swiss chard are foods with the most powerful immune-boosting and anticancer effects. Leafy greens are especially important because they contain an enormous amount of vitamins A, C, E, and K, minerals, and phytochemicals.

2. Walnuts: Rich in Mood-Boosting Omega-3 Fatty Acids

Walnuts are one of the richest plant sources of omega-3 fatty acids. Studies have revealed how omega-3 fatty acids support brain function and reduce depression symptoms.

3. Avocado: The Oleic Acid Gives You Brain Power

Avocados contain healthy fat that your brain needs in order to run smoothly. Three-fourths of the calories of an avocado are from fat, mostly monounsaturated fat, in the form of oleic acid. An average avocado contains 4 grams of protein and is filled with vitamin K, various forms of vitamin B (B9, B6, and B5), vitamin C, and vitamin E12.

4. Berries: Full of Cell-Repairing Antioxidants

Blueberries, raspberries, strawberries, and blackberries are some of the highest antioxidant foods available to us. I add a variety of these delicious fruits into my protein smoothies for my lunch. Antioxidants are designed to repair your cells and help prevent us from getting cancer and other illnesses.

5. Mushrooms: Helpful Tools to Lower Blood Sugar

The chemical properties in mushrooms oppose insulin, which helps lower blood sugar levels, evening out your mood. Mushrooms are also like a probiotic in that they promote healthy gut bacteria.

6. Onions: Layered With Cancer-Fighting Allium

Onions and all allium vegetables have been associated

with a decreased risk of several cancers. Allium vegetables are garlic, leeks, chives, shallots, and spring onions.

7. Tomatoes: Packed With Depression Fighting Ninjas

Tomatoes contain lots of folic acid and alpha-lipoic acid which are good for fighting depression. In most clinical of the studies, about one-third of depression patients were deficient in folate.

8. Beans: Satisfyingly High in Mood-Stabilizing Fiber

Beans digest slowly, which help stabilizes blood sugar levels. Beans are a starch that is not only full of fiber can help you with food cravings for bread and other processed grains. One of my favorite comfort and satisfying foods is my vegetarian chili with red kidney beans and black beans.

9. Seeds: Small but Mighty Sources of Omega-3s

Flaxseeds, hemp seeds, and chia seeds are especially good for your mood because they are rich in omega-3 fatty acids. I enjoy adding hemp and flax seeds into my salads. The fat in seeds increases the absorption of protective nutrients in vegetables eaten at the same meal.

10. Apples: Ripe With Antioxidants and Fiber

An apple a day does keep the doctor away! Apples are high in antioxidants. Antioxidants help to prevent and repair oxidation damage and inflammation on the cellular level. Apples are also full of soluble fiber, which balances blood sugar swings. One of my favorite snacks is peanut butter on apple slices. I get my omega-3 fatty acid along with some fiber.

13 MY TOP 15 TIPS FOR WEIGHT LOSS!

1. DON'T EAT AFTER YOUR KIDS. I USED TO ALWAYS EAT MY SON'S PIZZA CRUST WHICH WAS AN EXTRA 100 CALORIES. I DON'T KNOW WHY LITTLE CHILDREN WON'T EAT THE CRUST. SMH

2. DON'T DRINK YOUR CALORIES: NO SUGARY DRINKS, SWEET TEA, COFFEE, AND SODA. CURB SUGAR CRAVINGS. DON'T CONSUME ARTIFICIAL SWEETENERS AS A LOW-CALORIE DRINK SUBSTITUTE FOR SUGAR. (IT WILL TAKE YOU OUT OF KETOSIS IF YOU ARE INTERMITTENT FASTING) KETOSIS IS A STATE WHERE THE BODY HAS LOW CARBOHYDRATE LEVELS WHICH CAUSES THE BLOOD SUGAR LEVELS TO DROP. IN KETOSIS, THE BODY BEGINS BREAKING DOWN FAT TO USE AS ENERGY. I USE TO CONSUME DAILY: A LARGE SWEET TEA FROM MCDONALD'S (WHICH IS 280 CALORIES).

3. Walk at least 10k steps daily.

4. Don't eat after 8 pm (if you do, only eat those foods under 50 calories to stay in fast mode)

5. Make sure to have a caloric deficit of at least 500 calories a day. Do not cheat on the weekends. If you are unsure about how many calories you should consume daily go to this website: https://www.calculator.net/calorie-calculator.html

6. Drink lots and lots of water especially in the mornings and before meals.

7. Treat yourself (not food related) when you reach milestone goals. For example, when you lose ten lbs., 20lbs, halfway meet your goal, and when you meet your goal.

8. Stay focused, motivated, and positive

9. Be proud of every pound you lose.

10. Don't just rely on the scale. Look at how you're losing inches and how your clothes fit better to stay motivated.

11. Stay consistent and move every day. (Walk, run swimming, at home no equipment exercise).

NO EXCUSE TO NOT MOVE UNLESS YOU ARE ILL.

12. GET A FITBIT APP AND COUNT YOUR CALORIES AND MACROS!

13. LEARN TO LOVE YOUR NEW BODY BY SPEAKING POSITIVELY ABOUT IT. DON'T BODY SHAME YOURSELF!

14. SAY SELF-AFFIRMATIONS AND/OR SPEAK ALOUD SCRIPTURE TO KEEP YOUR MIND AND SPIRIT STRONG.

15. REMEMBER, EAT TO LIVE, NOT LIVE TO EAT. REMEMBER YOUR "WHY?" IT'S ABOUT HEALTH, NOT WHAT THEY THINK YOUR WEIGHT LOSS GOAL SHOULD BE.

Chapter 13 Journal Questions

1. Which of the 15 tips do you plan on trying first? Why?

2. Which sugar-filled drink is your favorite? What steps will you take to reduce or cut off completely the consumption of this drink in your diet?

3. What can change about your daily routine, so that you can make sure that you walk at least 10K steps daily?

4. CREATE FIVE POSITIVE WEIGHT LOSS AFFIRMATIONS THAT YOU WILL SAY TO YOURSELF DAILY. I GIVE YOU THREE. AFFIRMATIONS.

   A. I AM READY TO LOSE WEIGHT.
   B. I AM IN CONTROL OF WHAT I EAT AND DRINK.
   C. I RESPECT MY BODY.
   D.
   E.

5. WHAT DO YOU PLAN TO DO TO INCREASE YOUR CONSUMPTION OF WATER DAILY?

14 LET YOUR HATERS BE YOUR MOTIVATORS

My family and friends were my biggest supporters at first. Some of them may have forgotten what I looked like before I put on 40 pounds. It had been four years since I was at my normal average weight.

Most of my family was supportive. My spouse even told me that I looked anorexic and that he didn't want me to get too skinny. He was not used to me being a size 2. When we started dating, I was more of a size 6-8. I told him that I didn't appreciate his insensitive comments. As a dancer I was already sensitive about my weight and being called anorexic wasn't appropriate. He apologized and said that he loved me unconditionally regardless of how much I weighed.

I mention this intimate conversation between

my husband and me because sometimes your spouse or significant other may not want you to gain or lose weight. It could be for personal reasons, or they could be insecure. They could be jealous of your weight loss. They could feel some type of way because you are attracting unwarranted and unwanted attention that they are not happy about. Sometimes our spouses are not used to change, and they could be afraid that your relationship may change in a negative way. Make sure to keep the lines of communication open as you start this journey. Maybe you can offer to work out together as a couple.

I had one former student say that I shouldn't get too much smaller or it would look like I was wasting away. I had a few students that would always try to get me to eat knowing good and well I was fasting. Or they would try to sabotage my good eating habits by always offering the crack that got me fat in the first place, desserts.

In this weight loss journey, I had to realize that friends and family may have meant well, but I couldn't allow their comments or judgments to deter me from my personal health and fitness goals. When friends would ask me what I did to lose the weight, I would simply say intermittent fasting, working out, and clean eating. Most people knew that I was a vegetarian who once a week partook in eating seafood, basically a pescatarian. They would react by saying that my diet, I consider it a lifestyle, was too restrictive for them. One person said that they knew someone who lost weight doing intermittent fasting as well, but they couldn't personally fast for that long period of time.

Just know that your weight loss journey is yours and yours alone. Not everyone is going to understand the commitment and dedication that it will take to lose the weight and to maintain it. You have to remember your "why" daily. Your "why" is your personal reason to get healthy. My "why" was that I wanted to lose 40 pounds so that I could hopefully no longer take my high blood pressure pills. I also wanted to overcome my addiction to sugar and hopefully help lower my chances of developing type 2 diabetes. I wanted to lose the weight so that I could feel comfortable in my own skin again. When I was overweight, I did not recognize myself in the mirror. I noticed that I stopped taking selfies because I no longer felt attractive. I wanted to get back to the size I was used to for the majority of my life.

When I turned 40, chile that was a wakeup call. My body's metabolism seemed to have died or gone into a coma. It didn't just "slow down". I no longer could eat the foods that I ate when I was in my twenties. At 42, I really have to be aware of the calories that I intake daily and exercise daily. I now have experienced firsthand what happens when I let myself go and stop caring about what I eat when I eat, and if and when I exercise.

I used to think of exercise as a chore. I have had to change my mindset and view exercise as an important part of my daily life. I have tried to find ways to make exercising fun by taking different forms of dance classes. I have also learned how to vary up my exercise routine whether it is at home or when I can make it to the gym.

At the end of the day, take every negative, insensitive, and rude comment and use it as your motivation. For whatever reason, they felt the need to say those comments. However, let those comments be the fire that ignites the desire to make positive changes in your life. DO NOT sulk or dwell too long on the negative. Look forward to reaching those goals and achieving those milestones that you set for yourself. Stay motivated by saying affirmations to yourself. Read scripture, pray, and meditate. But most of all stay active and never give up on yourself. You can do this! I believe that you can attain anything that you set your mind to do! Remember at the end of the day, do you boo!

KEEP A SUCCESS JOURNAL

I love journals, and I highly recommend them. The only rule with your journal is it all has to be positive.

1. Record weight loss successes
2. Make a note of positive comments you receive
3. Write about positive changes you've made
4. Note down any changes you notice in your body physically and the way you feel

I have created space for this journal so that you can look back at on the days where you don't feel positive or motivated. Reading your journal entries during those times will help you stay on track to meet your health and weight loss goals.

Your Success Journal

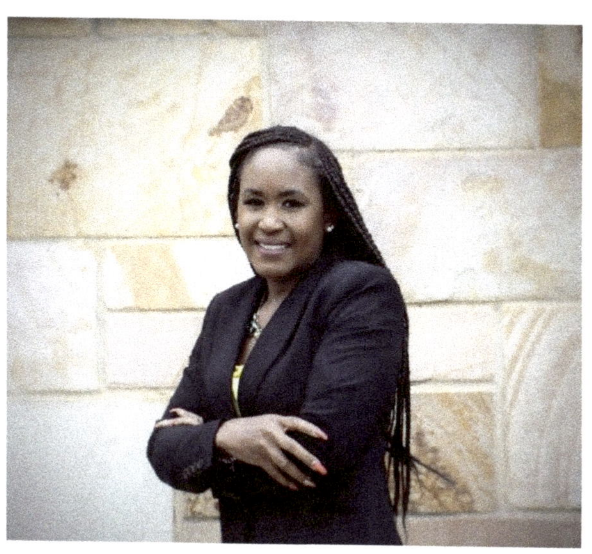

ABOUT THE AUTHOR

Tanae N. Walker is a wife and mother to seven children, three biological and four bonus. She is based out of North Carolina. She has been an educator for twelve years. When she hit her forties and gained over 45 pounds, she realized that she was going down a road that many of her family members have succumbed to. This road leads to obesity, high blood pressure, type 2 diabetes, even cancer. This book chronicles her journey losing 40 pounds, while over 40 and in just four months. In each chapter, she gives helpful, insightful, and relevant information to help you conceive, believe and achieve your health and weight loss goals.

You can connect with Tanae Walker on Facebook, Linkedin, Twitter @tanaewalker, and Instagram @tanaenwalker. You can also visit her website at www.tanaewalker.com.

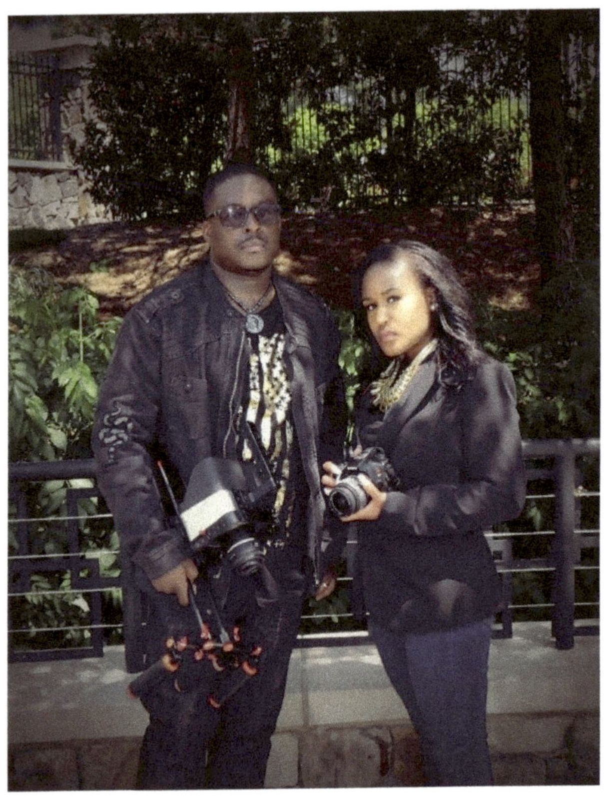

TNT Productions LLC was founded in 2014 by the power couple Todd and Tanae Walker. They work as a strong, effective, and efficient team to provide the services of photography and film for their clients. They spend endless hours editing, making sure that each and every photo will be a wonderful lasting memory to be enjoyed by their clients each and every time. When you book with TNT Productions LLC, you will get more than you paid for as far as professional customer service, quality photographs, and film.

Client Reviews:

As an artist I got what I was looking for to help promote...quick turnaround time, very professional, would be getting my business soon.
- Tre Da Songwriter Latter

~

Amazing photography! My senior pictures turned out better than imagined! I'd highly recommend TNT Productions for any of your photography needs.
-Karissa Ruiz

~

Awesome service! Extremely professional and dedicated to his ART!
-Princess Smith

~

I've been following TNT productions for a few years and I am always Blown Away with how creative they are! Absolutely perfect for wedding pictures because they will definitely capture the most majestic moments!!
-Raven Sykes

~

Was really awesome and loved the pictures. So professionally done and I would recommend others to get their pictures taken from this experience.
-Karina Baldwin

~

Definitely need to hit up TNT productions for your next video!
-Rook Mewsick

Been great working with you, throughout the movies, videos, etc! Keep up the good work!
-Allen Verde

Contact us:

Website:

www.tntproductions.net

Facebook:

TNT Productions & Photography
https://m.facebook.com/TNTProduction101

CPSIA information can be obtained
at www.ICGtesting.com
Printed in the USA
BVHW090158020619
549625BV00006B/8/P